BAPTISM THROUGH INCISION

Lam. 19.

H   fig.ᵃ 2ᵃ

I

G   N

M   L

O

fig.ᵃ 1ᵃ

B   A   B

BAPTISM THROUGH INCISION

The Postmortem Cesarean Operation in the Spanish Empire

Martha Few, Zeb Tortorici, and Adam Warren

The Pennsylvania State University Press
University Park, Pennsylvania

Library of Congress Cataloging-in-Publication Data

Names: Few, Martha, 1964– author. | Tortorici, Zeb, 1978– author. | Warren,
    Adam, Ph.D., author. | Arrese, Pedro José de, –1795. Rudimentos
    fisico-canonico-morales. English.
Title: Baptism through incision : the postmortem cesarean operation in the
    Spanish Empire / Martha Few, Zeb Tortorici, and Adam Warren.
Other titles: Latin American originals.
Description: University Park, Pennsylvania : The Pennsylvania State
    University Press, [2020] | Series: Latin American originals | Includes
    bibliographical references and index.
Summary: "Explores the history of the postmortem cesarean operation,
    which was performed in order to extract the fetus and save its soul
    through baptism. Examines accounts of the operation from across
    the Spanish empire in the eighteenth century"—Provided by
    publisher.
Identifiers: LCCN 2019056791 | ISBN 9780271086071 (paperback)
Subjects: LCSH: Arrese, Pedro José de, –1795. Rudimentos fisico-canonico-
    morales. | Cesarean section—Spain—History—18th century. |
    Cesarean section—Spain—Colonies—History—18th century. |
    Baptism—Catholic Church—History—18th century. | Medicine—
    Religious aspects—Catholic Church—History—18th century.
Classification: LCC RG761.F49 2020 | DDC 618.8/60946—dc23
LC record available at https://lccn.loc.gov/2019056791

We dedicate this book to our mothers:

Sue Ann Powell Fem
Roberta Bruno Tortorici
Susan Warren
Amina Hildegard Budde

CONTENTS

Latin American Originals (LAO) is a series of primary source texts on colonial Latin America. LAO volumes are accessible editions of texts translated into English—most of them for the very first time. Of the fifteen volumes now in print, nine illuminate aspects of the Spanish invasions in the Americas during the long century of 1494–1614, four push our understandings of the spiritual conquest and the early church in Spanish America in surprising directions, and the most recent two—including the present volume—take the series into exciting new territory.

Taken in the chronological order of their primary texts, *Of Cannibals and Kings* (LAO 7) comes first. It presents the earliest written attempts to describe Native American cultures, offering striking insight into how the first Europeans in the Americas struggled from the very start to conceive a "New World." *The Native Conquistador* (LAO 10) comes next, telling the story of the famous Spanish conquest expeditions into Mexico and Central America from 1519 to 1524—but from the startlingly different perspective of an Indigenous dynasty, with Ixtlilxóchitl, ruler of Tetzcoco, the alternative leading protagonist, as recounted by his great-great-grandson.

Next, chronologically, are LAO volumes 2, 1, and 9. *Invading Guatemala* shows how reading multiple accounts of conquest wars (in this case Spanish, Nahua, and Maya versions of the Guatemalan conflict of the 1520s) can explode established narratives and suggest a more complex and revealing conquest story. *Invading Colombia* challenges us to view the difficult Spanish invasion of Colombia in the 1530s as more representative of conquest campaigns than the better-known assaults on the Aztec and Inca Empires. It complements *The Improbable Conquest*, which presents letters written between 1537 and 1556 by Spaniards struggling—with a persistence that is improbable indeed—to found a colony along the hopefully named Río de la Plata.

Contesting Conquest (LAO 12) adds intriguingly to that trio, offering new perspectives on Nueva Galicia's understudied early history. Indigenous witnesses and informants, their voices deftly identified, selected, and presented, guide us through the grim, messy tale of repeated efforts there at conquest and colonization from the late 1520s through 1545. *The History of the New World* (LAO 11) offers the first English translation since 1847 of significant portions of a 1565 Italian book that, in its day, was a best seller in five languages. The merchant-adventurer Girolamo Benzoni mixed sharp observations and sympathy for Indigenous peoples with imaginary tales and wild history, influencing generations of early modern readers and challenging modern readers to sort out fact from fable.

The Conquest on Trial (LAO 3) features a fictional Indigenous embassy filing a complaint over the conquest in a court in Spain— the Court of Death. That text, the first theatrical examination of the conquest published in Spain, effectively condensed contemporary debates on colonization into one dramatic package. It contrasts well with *Defending the Conquest* (LAO 4), which presents a spirited, ill-humored, and polemic apologia for the Spanish conquest, written in 1613 by a lesser-known veteran conquistador.

LAO volumes 5, 6, 8, and 13 all explore aspects of Spanish efforts to implant Christianity in the Americas. Chronologically, *To Heaven or to Hell* (LAO 13) comes first, presenting the first complete English translation of a book by Bartolomé de Las Casas published in 1552— not his famous *Very Brief Account of the Destruction of the Indies* but his *Confessionary for Confessors*. The *Confessionary*'s less sensationalist content was eventually overshadowed by the *Very Brief Account* but initially was just as controversial and—to conquistadors and many other Spaniards—outrageously offensive in its demand that Spanish conquistadors, in effect, be themselves made subject to the spiritual conquest in the Americas.

Gods of the Andes (LAO 6) presents the first English edition of a 1594 manuscript describing Inca religion and the campaign to convert native Andeans. Its Jesuit author is surprisingly sympathetic to preconquest beliefs and practices, viewing them as preparing Andeans for the arrival of the faith from Spain. *Forgotten Franciscans* (LAO 5) casts new light on the spiritual conquest and the conflictive cultural world of the Inquisition in sixteenth-century Mexico. Both works expose wildly divergent views within the church in Spanish America—both on native religions and on how to replace them with Christianity. Complementing those two volumes by revealing the Indigenous side to the same process, *Translated Christianities* (LAO 8) presents religious texts translated from Nahuatl and Yucatec Maya. Designed to proselytize and ensure the piety of Indigenous parishioners, these texts show how such efforts actually contributed to the development of local Christianities, leading to fascinatingly multifaceted outcomes.

New directions for the series are opened up by the presentation in LAO 14 of the *Journal and History* of the Dutch expedition to Chile. *To the Shores of Chile* brings up to seven the number of languages from which LAO sources have been translated. It also extends the series into a new region of the Americas and forward into the 1640s, with a whole new perspective on European colonization, European-Indigenous interaction, and global competition in the age of empire.

The present volume takes the series even further forward in time. Using eighteenth-century Guatemala as their case study, Martha Few, Zeb Tortorici, and Adam Warren take us to one of the most fascinating intersections of faith and science in the early modern world. *Baptism Through Incision* is the first English publication—and the first expert presentation—of an eye-opening 1786 treatise on performing cesareans on pregnant women at the moment of their death. It explores anew many of the themes threaded through previous LAO volumes in the series: empire, salvation, the female body, and knowledge as an American battleground.

The source texts in LAO volumes are colonial-era rare books or archival documents, written in European or Mesoamerican languages. LAO authors are historians, anthropologists, and scholars of literature who have developed a specialized knowledge that allows them to locate, translate, and present these texts in a way that contributes to scholars' understanding of the period, while also making them readable for students and nonspecialists. Few, Tortorici, and Warren are such scholars, offering a stunning combination of skills, expertise, and knowledge that permits them to lend this series the benefit of their unique insights.

—Matthew Restall

ACKNOWLEDGMENTS

Collaborative research fellowships from the John Carter Brown
Library and the American Council of Learned Societies facilitated
the completion of this work and the development of a larger, ongo-
ing project on the history of the cesarean operation throughout the
Iberian World. We thank Neil Safier and the staff of the John Carter Brown Library, for making us feel welcome in Providence, and
Matthew Goldfeder and Cindy Mueller, for coordinating our ACLS
award. Support from the Department of Spanish and Portuguese
Languages and Literatures at New York University and the History
Departments at the Pennsylvania State University, the University of
Arizona, and the University of Washington made additional work on
the project possible. The authors especially acknowledge the gener-
osity of donors to these departments. These include Lenore Hanauer
and Howard and Frances Keller.

Numerous friends and colleagues provided expert support for this
project. Maternal and fetal-medicine specialist and OB-GYN Sameer
Gopalani offered advice on the contemporary cesarean section and
fetal survival inside the womb. Sandra Joshel shared knowledge
of Roman law and commented on fellowship applications. Marcos
Cueto and Susan Kellogg kindly wrote letters on our behalf. Leah
DeVun and Charity Urbanski generously translated Latin passages
for the introduction and chapter 1, respectively. Archivists and
librarians across the Americas, among them Thelma Porres of the
Centro de Investigaciones Regionales de Mesoamérica, directed us to
little-known sources. Two anonymous manuscript readers provided
invaluable comments. Sean Mannion and Susan Silver proved to be
outstanding copyeditors. Matthew Restall and Ellie Goodman have
enthusiastically supported this project since its inception.

The authors are especially grateful to Nina M. Scott, who gra-
ciously accepted our invitation and translated Arrese's difficult text

beautifully and from whom we learned a great deal about translation. Our own translations in chapter 2 build on that knowledge, though they pale in comparison to her work. Nina acknowledges in her translator's note several friends who assisted her with Latin and tricky Spanish phrases, whom we also thank.

Finally, we are grateful to our partners—Keisuke Hirano, Su Anne Takeda, and Scot Orriss—as well as our parents and families.

TRANSLATOR'S NOTE

Martha Few, Adam Warren, and Zeb Tortorici contacted me to do
the translation of the Arrese treatise in 2015. Principally a literary
scholar, I had done previous translations in literature and history and,
based on a quick reading of the document, thought I could do this
fairly easily. I was wrong.

Arrese specifically stated that he wanted to write "in a plain style,
suitable to common folk," but he led me down many linguistic and
conceptual labyrinths: interminable sentences, unclear or missing
antecedents, obscure vocabulary, erratic spelling and punctuation,
references to little-known clergy or scientists. Ferreting out their
identities and significance necessitated extra research.

What is there to do when sentences are just plain beyond one's
ability to translate? We go to friends and colleagues. Of particular
help were Asunción Lavrin, distinguished colonial historian, and
David Arbesú, a medievalist with an impressive grasp of arcane
language. Betsy Mathews and Christopher van den Berg helped with
the Latin.

My sincere thanks to them all.

Thanks also to the John Carter Brown Library for the collabo
rative grant to work together on this translation. Although it was
an exhausting and mind-stretching activity, it turned us into good
friends who sincerely appreciated a cold beer at the end of a long
workday.

—Nina M. Scott

Introduction

Postmortem Cesareans and Pedro José de Arrese's Guatemalan Treatise in Historical Context

MARTHA FEW, ZEB TORTORICI, AND ADAM WARREN

In October 1804 the newspaper *Gazeta de Guatemala* published a few lines describing a surgical procedure that may seem to readers today as strange and even macabre. The *gazeta* gave a brief yet explicit account of what is often called a *postmortem cesarean operation*—that is, a cesarean operation performed on a deceased pregnant woman—carried out in 1799 at a mission in the frontier Petén region of colonial Central America. A married Maya woman, Nicolasa Chatá, in advanced stages of pregnancy, lay dying of smallpox, with her husband, Marcos Cob, and the local Catholic priest by her side. As her condition worsened, the priest called on an unidentified barber-surgeon, "an Indian who had been instructed in the necessary procedures," to prepare to carry out the operation on Chatá immediately upon her death. The priest's goal was decidedly not to save the life of the fetus but rather to save its soul by baptizing it during its brief moments of life after being surgically extracted from the deceased mother's womb. Knowing that she would not survive the smallpox, Chatá allegedly "begged" that the procedure be performed on her body. The barber-surgeon gathered the needed medical instruments and, at the moment of her death, surgically opened Chatá's uterus (through the side of her belly, as instruction manuals such as Pedro José de Arrese's advised) under the priest's supervision and removed the fetus. The priest then baptized it, but only after judging

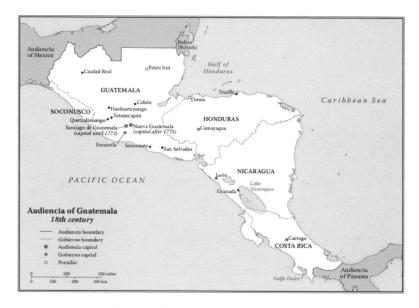

MAP 1 Audiencia of Guatemala with significant locations marked. Drawn by Scott Zillmer, XNR Productions. Commissioned by Martha Few. © 2014 Martha Few.

"with certainty" that it was alive. The fetus quickly died, however, and was buried together with Chatá in consecrated ground. The priest then recorded this rather unique instance of an *entierro doble* (double burial) in his parish death registry.[1]

Over the course of the twentieth century, the cesarean operation became an increasingly common procedure employed on living women to facilitate a nonvaginal birth, from which both the woman and the fetus were fully expected to recover. Indeed, some readers of this volume likely were born by cesarean. In the eighteenth century, however, this was not the case, and the operation was performed almost exclusively on women already deceased. News of the case of Chatá, much like other recorded postmortem cesarean operations in this period, was not published for the purpose of generating an emotional reaction among readers and did not on its own elicit any particular response on the part of colonial authorities. At the same time, this particular operation was noteworthy enough to publicize

1. *Gazeta de Guatemala*, October 1, 1804, 453–54.

in the *Gazeta de Guatemala* in a series of articles that also included practical instructions and medical-religious justifications. Taken together, these works constituted a clear effort to inspire others to perform cesareans on deceased pregnant women in similar situations. Such journalistic acts of documenting and disseminating successful cesareans thus shed light on how members of the church, government officials, and ordinary people sought to transform understandings of life and death, salvation, and the female body through the introduction and adoption of an extraordinary surgical procedure. Furthermore, when juxtaposed with other texts from Guatemala and across the Spanish Empire included in this volume, they reveal variations in how everyday people in distinct settings understood, engaged with, and ascribed meaning to this procedure through its application and rejection.

In colonial Guatemala, where Chatá's postmortem cesarean took place, these efforts began in 1785, when the Audiencia of Guatemala's president enacted a law mandating postmortem cesareans for all deceased pregnant women and even those *suspected* of being pregnant when they had passed away.[2] That same year Guatemala's archbishop issued an edict in support of the mandate, excommunicating from the Catholic Church the pregnant woman's family members and any other bystanders if a postmortem cesarean had not been carried out immediately after her death. While numerous texts on the operation and fetal baptism had been published in Spain and elsewhere in years prior, eventually reaching Guatemala among the further reaches of the Spanish empire, members of Guatemala's own elite pushed for these policies. And so, when King Charles IV of Spain enacted the 1804 royal order mandating the postmortem procedure in all of Spain's dominions, the Audiencia of Guatemala and other regions in colonial Latin America already had such laws because of the efforts of local political and religious elites.[3]

Postmortem cesareans were part of the relatively new project of the colonial state's direct intervention into subject populations' physical health and well-being, a project that also included formal

2. The Audiencia of Guatemala was a royal court that exercised jurisdiction over what is today Guatemala, Honduras, El Salvador, Belize, Nicaragua, Costa Rica, and the Mexican state of Chiapas.

3. On the 1804 royal order, see Rigau-Pérez, "Surgery at the Service of Theology."

medical campaigns to control smallpox, typhus, measles, and other epidemic diseases.[4] Authorities introduced new technologies of first inoculation and then vaccination for the prevention of smallpox, and medical physicians advocated for urban hygiene and sanitation measures based on how they understood disease to be produced and transmitted. Equally important, however, postmortem cesareans were also an extension of centuries-old baptism and religious-conversion campaigns that aimed to ensure the spiritual health and salvation of the *audiencia*'s colonial populations, especially Indigenous people, who were legally defined as new to Catholicism and thus requiring instruction. This came, by the end of the eighteenth century, to include fetuses and their souls, which were thought to need cleansing of Adam and Eve's original sin to reach heaven; otherwise, they would reside in limbo. Performing cesareans on deceased female bodies for fetal baptism was thus a product of both medical and theological debates that took place throughout the empire as well as at the local level. The operation was intended to serve spiritual ends along with the larger goal of maintaining and propagating an empire managed by ruling elites, in part, by trying to ensure that the souls of colonized subjects' infants would be eternally brought into the fold of Catholicism.

Knowledge about cesarean operations quickly became part of the new ideas and scientific and medical advancements circulating broadly among transatlantic Enlightenment cultures. Guatemala president José de Estachería's 1786 decree reflected the desire of audiencia elites not only to proceed correctly on traditional political and religious grounds but also to stand with other "modern" nations: "The cesarean procedure, which removes the fetus [*feto*] from dead women with an incision, is established in this Kingdom [of Guatemala] not only because of its humanitarian and religious uses but also because it is recommended by all the political rights observed in all the political nations."[5] The president's argument here is that all fetuses, regardless of what other colonial categories they fit into, deserved baptism when the woman, for whatever reason, could not

---

4. For more on the connection between Enlightenment-era antiepidemic campaigns and efforts to spread the postmortem cesarean operation, see Few, *For All of Humanity*, chap. 3, "Constructing Colonial Fetuses."

5. "Operación cesária," 1785, A1.22-1509-x, Archivo General de Centro América (hereafter cited as AGCA), fol. 114v.

carry the pregnancy to term. In the process a woman's uterus became at once a contested political, religious, and medicalized space, much as it is in struggles over reproductive rights today. It was the independent object of surveillance and surgical intervention performed by a parish priest and an Indigenous barber-surgeon (as in the case of Chatá) or by colonial politicians, local surgeons, and other professional and religious men in colonial society. The woman herself lost importance in the legislation, except as a body on whom intervention was required and as someone whose behavior when alive might threaten the physical and spiritual health of the fetus inside her. As Martha Few argues, the fetus was constructed as a "colonial subject" at the intersection of eighteenth-century society, the spread of new Enlightenment doctrines of governance, the continuing power of the church, and the emergence of medicine that targeted the health of colonial populations.[6]

As becomes clear over the course of the late colonial period, while the fetus's physical survival was certainly desired, the overarching goal of the postmortem cesarean operation was to ensure the fetus's place in heaven through the sacrament of baptism. Depictions of reproduction, childbirth, surgical intervention, life, death, and salvation spread in late colonial society not only through legislation but also through multiple texts, such as Pedro José de Arrese's *Rudimentos físico, canónico, morales . . . Sobre el bautismo de fetos abortivos y operación cesárea en las mugeres que mueren embarazadas (Physical, Canonical, Moral Principles . . . on the Baptism of Miscarried Fetuses and the Cesarean Operation on Women Who Die Pregnant)*, published in 1786 in Guatemala and translated into English for the first time in this volume.

Old World Origins and Influences

How might we trace the origins of Arrese's treatise and explain its appearance in the final decades of Spanish colonial rule? Arrese's work did not come about in a vacuum, and the ideas presented in it were not exclusively his own. Rather, his treatise forms part of a longer genealogy of eighteenth-century texts through which knowledge

6. Few, *For All of Humanity*, 131–32.

of obstetrics, miscarriage, the postmortem cesarean operation, and fetal baptism spread from Europe across the Spanish Empire, reaching not just the Americas but also the Philippines, which had been colonized by Spain in the mid-sixteenth century and was formally incorporated into the Viceroyalty of New Spain in 1565. These works transformed the role of priests, surgeons, and midwives by exhorting them to learn and perform the cesarean operation, and the texts resulted in new legislation requiring such training and the procedure's use on women like Chatá. Yet these eighteenth-century texts clearly had much longer European genealogies, though the exact origins of the cesarean operation are impossible to pinpoint.

Some of the earliest-known texts that explicitly broach the cesarean operation were authored in the ancient and early medieval worlds. Scholars, for example, have uncovered scant references to the operation having been performed in 715 BCE, when the Roman king Numa Pompilius proclaimed the *lex regia*, stating that "royal law denies a woman (who has died pregnant) to be buried before the child is cut out from her, which will be done against hope of reviving when the pregnant woman seems to be dead." Similarly succinct references appear in ancient Indian and Roman as well as medieval Jewish and Islamic texts.[7] One of the earliest medieval European texts to explicitly discuss the postmortem cesarean operation was the early fourteenth-century *Lilium medicinae* by Bernard de Gordon (1270–1330), written by a French doctor and professor of medicine at the University of Montpellier, though his text was not officially printed until the late fifteenth century in the cities of Naples, Lyons, and Venice. For centuries, then, mention of the cesarean operation in published works was sporadic at best.

The authoring of de Gordon's work anticipated a gradual increase in the dissemination of knowledge about the procedure that took place over the fourteenth century. As historian Maaike van der Lugt notes, "Postmortem fetal excisions were not originally considered part of medicine. Evidence for the involvement of barbers and surgeons appears only in the fourteenth century. By this time, some learned physicians and surgeons had also started to describe the procedure, despite its absence in ancient and Arabic medical sources—a

---

7. Cited in the original Latin by Blumenfeld-Kosinski, *Not of Woman Born*, 164n48. Arrese himself references Numa's law; see also pages 21–24.

reflection of Christian concerns, new social demands and the growing medicalization of childbirth."[8] During this period French physician and surgeon Guy de Chauliac (1300–1368) wrote about the postmortem cesarean in his treatise on learned surgery, the *Inventarium sive Chirurgia magna*, which he completed in 1363 and which was translated from Latin into English, French, Hebrew, Italian, Dutch, and Provençal, a dialect of Occitan once spoken in southern France.[9] As Katharine Park notes, by the later fourteenth and early fifteenth centuries, the postmortem cesarean had become a familiar presence in medical treatises "and was often [visually] depicted in illustrated histories of the Roman Empire in connection with the birth of Julius Caesar."[10]

Although these early texts were not dedicated entirely to the cesarean operation, they discussed the operation's importance in the broader context of questions surrounding physical and moral health. As such, the texts embed their discussions of the procedure, and the imperative to perform it, in a wider discussion of anatomy, fractures, dislocations, wounds, complicated pregnancies, ulcers, tumors, and a range of other medical and surgical issues. In addition, in the late sixteenth and early seventeenth centuries postmortem dissections and operations were increasingly performed on the bodies of women and men considered for sainthood—yet another manifestation of the intricate and intimate relationality of science and religion.[11]

Especially in Spain, the sixteenth century saw a proliferation of surgical manuals that discussed the postmortem cesarean operation in one way or another. Among these works were texts such as Luis Lobera de Ávila's 1551 *Libro del regimen de la salud y de la esterilidad de los hombres y mujeres* (Book on the regimen of health and on sterility in men and women) and Rodrigo de Castro's 1603 *Tratado sobre las enfermedades de las mujeres* (Treatise on the sicknesses of women), as well as the 1658 theological treatise penned by Catholic priest Jerónimo Florentino, titled *De Hominibus dubiis sive de baptismo abortivorum* (On doubtful humans or the baptism of

8. Van der Lugt, "Formed Fetuses and Healthy Children," in Hopwood, Flemming, and Kassell, *Reproduction*, 172.

9. See Caulhiaco, *Inventarium sive Chirurgia Magna*.

10. Park, "Managing Childbirth and Fertility," in Hopwood, Flemming, and Kassell, *Reproduction*, 160.

11. Bouley, *Pious Postmortems*.

miscarriages).[12] None, however, devoted attention to the theological arguments for the cesarean operation's use in combination with fetal baptism in the way that Arrese and those authors who most directly influenced him would later do. Indeed, in their eighteenth-century works, the procedure and the accompanying baptismal ritual were the exclusive focus and formed part of a larger colonial campaign to save souls.

These medicoreligious treatises, and eventually the corresponding legislation, on the postmortem cesarean operation that spread throughout Europe, the Americas, and beyond relied in great part on scientific developments in Europe that enabled embryos to be seen for the first time and fetuses to be observed in new ways. Advances included, for example, the use of a single-lensed microscope to view microbial life in Europe from the 1670s on and, in the mid- to late 1700s, new methods to discern visually the rhythmic movements of the fetus within a woman's womb in what eventually came to be known as the field of embryology.[13] Hence, the title of one key book, *Sacred Embryology* (*Embryologia sacra*), deliberately merges religious fervor with the scientific study of the development of the fetus. We also see this focus on the fetus's visibility clearly in Arrese's text when, for instance, he writes that on the third day after conception, "one can already see something like a little worm with a head; in this, as well as in the trunk, one can, with the aid of a microscope, detect the components of a human body."

Such scientific advancement and incursions into the human body also engendered new moral quandaries. A notable feature of debates throughout the early modern period and leading up to the mid-eighteenth century is their focus on when the cesarean operation should be used and whether it should be performed on living women to save the life of the fetus. Although this is something that later authors like Arrese discouraged, Valencian doctor Jaime Alcalá y Martínez wrote about performing a cesarean on a live woman in an excerpt of his 1753 *Dissertación médico-chirúrgica sobre una operación cesárea, executada en muger, y feto vivos en esta ciudad de Valencia* (Medical-surgical dissertation about a cesarean operation, carried

---

12. Demerson, "Cesárea *post mortem*."
13. For more on viewing technologies and the role rhythm played in the evolution of embryology, see Wellmann, *Form of Becoming*.

out on a live woman and fetus in this city of Valencia), translated
and included in chapter 2. Paula de Demerson notes that Alcalá y
Martínez's actions were censured as being criminal in nature.[14]
    The doctor was not unique, however; there is evidence that other
surgeons and medical doctors practiced the operation on live women
in the Kingdom of Portugal as well as in other parts of Spain. Diverse
eighteenth-century writings about midwifery—instructing women
on how to be efficacious *comadres* or *parteras* (midwives)—and
on the nascent field of obstetrics, published in several European
languages, also broached the topic of the cesarean operation.[15] For
instance, Dr. Sebastián Melli's *La comadre instruida en su oficio*
(The midwife instructed in her craft), published first in Venice in
1721, discussed the operation's usefulness for women both living
and dead. The German surgeon Martín Schurigio, in his *Embrio-
logia histórico-médica* (Historical-medical embryology), published
in Dresden in 1732, dedicated a chapter in support of the practice,
though not everyone agreed.[16] For example, in his 1756 *Nuevo y
natural modo de auxiliar a las mujeres en los lances peligrosos de los
partos* (New and natural way to aid women during dangerous events
in childbirth), Babil de Gárate y Casabona, surgeon from the city of
Pamplona, critiqued the practice of performing a cesarean operation
on women either living or dead, instead advising readers to insert a
syringe with baptismal waters into the uterus of the dying woman
to confer the sacrament on the soon-to-expire fetus. Arrese briefly
touches on this use of the syringe in his text, although—citing the
work of French obstetrician François Mauriceau (1637–1709), whom
he refers to throughout as "Francisco Morisó"—he expresses some
reservations about performing fetal baptism by this means.
    Readers of Arrese's *Physical, Canonical, Moral Principles* will
note that he engages two key authors from the mid-eighteenth
century—the Spanish Antonio José Rodríguez and the Italian Francesco Cangiamila—and incorporates examples from their works into
his own discussions. Both were friars, as were several others who
published on the cesarean operation and fetal baptism. This made

14. Demerson, "Cesárea *post mortem*," 189.
15. *Partera* means midwife, defined by the *Diccionario de autoridades* as "the
woman that in her profession assists she who is giving birth, commonly called the
comadre" (vol. 5).
16. Martín Schurigio is also known as Martin Schurig.

the cesarean operation movement one inextricably linked to shifting understandings of life, death, the soul, and salvation within the church. Rodríguez's and Cangiamila's texts first appeared in print, respectively, in the Spanish city of Zaragoza and in Palermo, on the island of Sicily, which at the time formed part of Spain's territorial possessions. Rodríguez, a Spanish Cistercian monk, published *Nuevo aspecto de teología médico-moral* (New aspect of medical-moral theology) in 1742, while Cangiamila, a Sicilian friar who later was appointed inquisitor, published *Sacred Embryology* in 1745. Although the latter text was in Italian and Latin, it was quickly translated into Spanish and several other European languages. Multiple editions of both Cangiamila's and Rodríguez's texts were published between the 1740s and the 1780s. In the case of Rodríguez's text, later editions incorporated substantial changes.

Both Cangiamila and Rodríguez built on medical and obstetrical knowledge produced throughout Europe in the sixteenth, seventeenth, and eighteenth centuries, though occasionally much earlier as well. Their books reflected the ways in which information about pregnancy and childbirth circulated among eighteenth-century authors, resulting in a complex matrix of knowledge and misinformation concerning the female body under an increasingly male medical gaze. Cangiamila's text proved especially influential, perhaps more so than the work of Rodríguez, as readers beyond Sicily and the Italian peninsula quickly gained access to it through printings in multiple languages. Building on earlier works and engaging his contemporaries, Cangiamila argued at length that carrying out the operation to baptize and save the souls of the unborn was a fundamental duty of priests, surgeons, and midwives. He also made crucial theological arguments about when the fetus becomes ensouled, disputed claims that priests should not be allowed to perform surgery on women's bodies, and refuted the concept of limbo as the destiny of those who died unbaptized.

Perhaps most important, his work decried what he saw as the high rate of voluntary and involuntary miscarriages—which he termed *abortos*—among women of various social and class backgrounds, as well as the practice of infanticide. Such moral panic around the topics of miscarriage, abortion, and infanticide are also regularly reflected in eighteenth-century medical treatises from Spain and its colonies (though, perhaps paradoxically, there are relatively few criminal cases of either abortion or infanticide for places like colonial Mexico and Guatemala). Yet, as Nora Jaffary in her work on childbirth and contraception in late colonial and early national Mexico points out, popular practices around the consumption of herbs and remedies to either provoke, regulate, or detain the menses, childbirth, or afterbirth often greatly diverged from official proscriptions: "Colonial Mexicans considered provoking the menses to be legally and socially acceptable, while Mexican legal and medicinal authorities viewed providing or receiving intentional abortions [by any means] as both unlawful and immoral."[17] By narrating lurid stories of "ignorant" mothers who either deliberately induced a miscarriage or killed their newborn children—stories that likely bore no relation to the actual behavior of women in Sicily—Cangiamila argued that priests were required to prevent and reform such behavior. Reflecting an obsession with these concerns, he stressed the need to police pregnancies, identify women who might be concealing a pregnancy, ensure that women who died were not pregnant, and perform the operation on those who did die pregnant for the purpose of baptizing the fetus. Indeed, he provided clear instructions for the operation and described several variations in the practice of baptism that should be allowed, building on centuries of theological debate about the ritual's proper use.

Rodríguez's *Nuevo aspecto* included similar arguments about miscarriage and infanticide as well as the need to employ cesareans to save the souls of unborn fetuses imperiled by pregnant women's deaths. In later revised editions Rodríguez added substantially to the original work, pulling examples from Cangiamila's text and debating him. For example, Rodríguez drew on Cangiamila's writings when discussing whether the cesarean operation should be performed on living women, and he cited examples from Cangiamila of miscarriages and instances when the operation was performed on deceased women. Perhaps most important, Rodríguez criticized Cangiamila for stealing his thunder. Noting that *Nuevo aspecto* was published several years before *Sacred Embryology*, Rodríguez resented the attention the Sicilian friar's work received and believed his own book deserved greater credit.

---

17. Jaffary, *Reproduction and Its Discontents*, 81.

Both Rodríguez's and Cangiamila's texts differed from the medieval and early modern studies of the cesarean operation on which they were based by championing the procedure as a spiritual and political obligation for priests and others. In this sense their works, beyond contributing to surgical knowledge and theological debates about the soul, came to have political ramifications through the development of broader policies. For example, they prompted Charles III to issue a *pragmática* (decree) on August 9, 1749, which was approved by Pope Benedict XIV, requiring the operation and the baptism of the unborn in the Kingdom of Sicily.[18] The *pragmática* appears to have been built on local legislation already approved in Sicily and was translated into other languages for dissemination to other Catholic countries. The Spanish Crown and its authorities issued other edicts and decrees on the issue well into the first half of the nineteenth century, as new works on the cesarean operation appeared in print. One such decree was the aforementioned one issued in Guatemala in 1785, which prompted the operation's use on women like Chatá. Many of these pieces of legislation were read and posted in town squares throughout the empire.

Cesarean Texts in the Broader Spanish Empire

In the Spanish colonies Cangiamila's and Rodríguez's works resulted in the publication of new texts in the second half of the eighteenth century that sought to introduce the operation and the practice of fetal baptism in a colonial context. In what ways did these texts differ, both from the works of these European authors and one another? In Mexico City, the capital of the Viceroyalty of New Spain, two texts appeared in print by the mid-1770s that lifted and translated long passages from Cangiamila. One of them, Ignacio Segura's *Avisos saludables a las parteras para el cumplimiento de su obligación* (Healthful advice for midwives for the fulfillment of their obligation), sought to transform portions of Cangiamila's writings into a practical set of instructions for midwives, whom the author believed must learn to carry out the cesarean operation in case a surgeon or priest was not present to perform it. Portions of Segura's text are

18. Rigau-Pérez, "Surgery at the Service of Theology," 385.

included in translation in chapter 2. The second and more widely circulated text was Friar José Manuel Rodríguez's *La caridad del sacerdote para con los niños encerrados en el vientre de sus madres difuntas* (The charity of the priest for children enclosed in the belly of their deceased mothers), to which Segura refers interested readers at the end of *Avisos saludables*. Rodríguez's work, published in 1772, included alongside the main text copies of letters from Viceroy Antonio María Bucareli y Ursúa, the highest government authority in New Spain, that circulated from town to town in 1772 to instruct justices and other officials to order postmortem cesareans and baptism and to fine those who refused to allow it. Rodríguez also included a letter from Archbishop Alonso Núñez de Haro y Peralta, the viceroyalty's highest religious authority, who, citing Charles III's 1749 *pragmática*, instructed priests of all kinds to keep a copy of José Manuel Rodríguez's book on hand so that they could carry out the operation if needed. Priests were also to ensure that several persons in each town and village received instruction in the operation and agreed to perform it when required. The priests were to offer eighty days of indulgences to those who carried it out.[19]

A text framed in a substantially different, more urgent tone appeared in Peru later in the eighteenth century. In 1781, during a massive set of largely Indigenous uprisings in the Andes that threatened to end Spanish colonial rule, Friar Francisco González Laguna published in Lima *El zelo sacerdotal para con los niños no-nacidos* (Priestly zeal for the unborn children). As Adam Warren demonstrates, while González Laguna was not unique in drawing on Cangiamila's work, he differed from other authors in seeking to adapt the Sicilian friar's arguments and sense of urgency to the local context of rebellion. He framed his text with a description of a battle in Upper Peru (present-day Bolivia), which is translated and included in chapter 2 of this volume. During the battle Indigenous rebels allegedly slaughtered pregnant women and cut open their bellies to kill the unborn fetuses, thereby depriving them of salvation. Recounting how a parish priest had entered the battlefield to baptize the exposed fetuses until he himself was killed, González Laguna argued that postmortem cesareans and fetal baptism were part of a

---

19. An indulgence is when a pope or a priest grants a remission of the punishment for sin to shorten one's time in purgatory.

larger campaign against the work of the devil and the alleged barbarism of Indigenous colonial subjects. For him they became tools enabling priests to evangelize and teach Indigenous people by pious example. González Laguna's depiction of Indigenous people in the Andes, which Warren reconstructs, thus stands in sharp contrast with later accounts of Chatá and her husband in Guatemala, who allowed and even requested the operation, and the Indigenous barber-surgeons who performed it on Chatá and others for the purpose of baptizing the unborn. Archival records shed light on rebels' actions and motives and lead us to question González Laguna's account of this episode of violence and salvation in Upper Peru. Nevertheless, the account caused Peru's viceroy, Agustín de Jáuregui, to enact a published edict or mandate, known as a *bando*, to require the operation and fetal baptism. The document was read in 1781 in Lima's town square, according to the protocol and usage of war.[20]

Arrese's *Physical, Canonical, Moral Principles* first appeared in print in 1786 (with a listed publication date of December 1785) in a context very different from that of the war-torn Peruvian Andes. Colonial Guatemala certainly was not in a state of war, and while it constituted an important part of Spain's overseas territories and a key site for the church's evangelizing mission because of its large Indigenous Maya populations, it was more peripheral in an economic and political sense. The absence of war in Guatemala and its presence in Peru also shaped a key distinction between Arrese's and González Laguna's texts. The former was structured as a question-and-answer dialogue, which would have been accessible to a wide audience of potential practitioners, even those located in the most remote villages and missions of Guatemala, while González Laguna's work included denser prose and was directed primarily at priests and other learned men charged with bringing this procedure to remote, "barbaric" regions of Peru. In this sense González Laguna saw priests as engaging in a spiritual war for the salvation of the unborn, while Arrese believed that the project of saving souls through fetal baptism could potentially be carried out by any "rational" member of colonial society in Guatemala: men and women, laypeople and religious, midwives, barber-surgeons, and others.

20. For more on González Laguna, see Warren, "Operation for Evangelization."

Ultimately, however, Arrese's work was similar to González Laguna's in that it also sought to adapt the teachings of Cangiamila and Rodríguez to a local colonial context. For example, Arrese argued that Cangiamila's perceptions of robust, strong rural women in Sicily did not correspond to his own perceptions of the rural women of Guatemala. Drawing on racial stereotypes of Indigenous people, he believed that they were more fragile than their European counterparts. This is why Arrese cites the early seventeenth-century Spanish theologian Antonio de Quintana Dueñas on the point that pregnant women in general need not fast or abstain from meat since they need more food and nutrition for the fetus, a point he sees as especially pertinent to Guatemala. Arrese adamantly expressed that "these and other moral opinions written in Europe and based on physical and experimental reasons are not generally adaptable to our countries because the reasons themselves as well as our climates are so different. Over here [in Guatemala] being a woman from the country does not mean that she is robust, and one finds perhaps as much frailty and delicate health in the country as in the cities." Arrese thus expresses the notion that the climate in Guatemala—and throughout the Americas in general—was inferior to that of Europe, which negatively affected the health and well-being of its Indigenous inhabitants especially.

González Laguna made similar arguments about the condition and health of Spanish and enslaved African women on Peru's coast, in addition to offering observations about the health and behavior of Indigenous women in Peru's highlands. As such, both his text and Arrese's formed part of a much larger movement—which would continue in the decades to follow—in which the cesarean operation and fetal baptism became part of the Crown's and the church's colonial mission. Indeed, Charles IV's universal 1804 edict required postmortem cesareans and fetal baptism throughout Spain's colonies. In this way colonial decrees sought to establish consistent practices with regard to saving the souls of the unborn, while figures like Arrese sought to adapt the teaching of such practices to local and regional settings.

Arrese and the Guatemalan Context

Few details of Arrese's life and career can be found in the archives. We do not know when he was born, though we do know that he died on January 5, 1795, in the audiencia's capital, Nueva Guatemala. We also know that he was an ordained priest and that he was permitted to live and work in the capital in the service of the *curia diocesana*—that is, a group of persons who assist the bishop of that diocese. At the time that Arrese published his cesarean operation manual with the printing press run by the "widow of Sebastián de Arévalo" in 1786, he was working as a *promotor fiscal* for the archbishopric and as secretary to Archbishop Cayetano Francos y Monroy.[21] The postmortem cesarean operation came to the attention of the archbishop and audiencia president José de Estachería in the mid-1780s from the surgeon Toribio Carabajal. Around the same time that Arrese penned his cesarean operation manual, Estachería commissioned three medical doctors from the University of San Carlos in Nueva Guatemala to write simple step-by-step instructions for confirming maternal death and performing the procedure to extract the fetus.[22] A translated excerpt of these medical instructions is included in chapter 2.

Concern for practical and scientific information about pregnancy, miscarriages, and childbirth was not limited to colonial officials or to women. An interested, literate public in this Enlightenment era eagerly consumed news of medical innovations and therapies as well as new ideas of the day for treating difficult births and preventing miscarriages. Colonial Central America's first printing house was established in 1660 in the capital city of Santiago de Guatemala.[23] Others followed in the seventeenth and eighteenth centuries, publishing the work of Guatemala's intellectuals as well as translations of important foreign authors; these works included postmortem

21. Lanning, *Eighteenth-Century Enlightenment*, 260. A *promotor fiscal* was a prosecuting officer (in ecclesiastical, inquisitorial, or diocesan courts) trained in civil and canon law.

22. "Despacho del sup[eri]or gobierno para que se haga practicar la operación cesárea," February 16, 1786, A1-6098-55547, AGCA, fols. 1r–17v. The commissioned doctors were José Flores, José de Córdova, and Manuel Merlo. The instructions were copied by hand and sent to all the major towns and hamlets in colonial Central America.

23. The capital city of the Audiencia of Guatemala shifted in 1773 from Santiago de Guatemala to Nueva Guatemala after a destructive earthquake.

cesarean manuals. The University of San Carlos, established in 1680 and also located in Guatemala's capital, produced a small but influential number of Guatemalan-born scientists and medical doctors, both laypeople and priests, during the eighteenth century. Not only did the university provide a corps of science and agriculture professionals, but its graduates—1,300 from 1775 to 1821—formed a key sector of the public that bought, read, and wrote for the paper media at the time.[24]

Given this interest in Enlightenment medical cultures in colonial Guatemala and in Europe, why would a postmortem cesarean be left in the hands of an Indigenous barber-surgeon, as in the case of Chatá? Successful colonization also depended in part on the ability of colonial officials to form alliances with Indigenous elites and others, such as Indigenous barber-surgeons, to maintain order, transmit Spanish cultural and medical practices, and promote Christianity among the colonized peoples. The description of Chatá's cesarean does not characterize the surgical extraction of her fetus as exceptional, however. In fact, this barber-surgeon is merely mentioned, without any further description. Unlike some of the other men in this narrative, including Chatá's husband and the priest who performed another of the cesareans that season, his name is never included.

Indigenous men also performed postmortem cesareans elsewhere in New Spain. Historian Rosemary Keupper Valle documented fourteen cesareans carried out between 1799 and 1826 in Alta California (now largely the state of California), and Indigenous men at the Mission San José performed two of them. In December 1825 Narciso and Silvestre, both described as "Indian," together performed a postmortem cesarean under the supervision of Friar Narciso Durán. In March 1829 the same Indigenous man Narciso performed another alone at the Mission San José, again supervised by the same priest.[25] As these examples show, that an Indigenous barber-surgeon in Guatemala would perform postmortem cesareans was not completely exceptional—nor was the figure of the Indigenous healer in colonial society. The Maya and other pre-Columbian Mesoamerican peoples

24. Dym, "Conceiving Central America," in Paquette, *Enlightened Reform*, 105.
25. No surnames were given for the Indigenous cesarean performers Narciso and Silvestre. See Valle, "Cesarean Operation."

had well-developed medical cultures with a sophisticated range of healing specialists of all genders. Maya women in many cases acted as midwives who specialized in treating women and their fetuses through pregnancy, childbirth, and the postpartum period.[26] After the conquest period, despite Christianization campaigns and the shock of mass deaths from epidemic disease, Indigenous communities continued to reproduce socially an adapted and transformed medical tradition, and Indigenous medical specialists passed on medical knowledge and trained the next generation of healers and midwives.

Extant sources from the colonial period on Maya conceptualizations of the fetus provide only brief and partial glimpses of this complicated issue. One way Maya ideas about the fetus came into the historical record was through depictions of magical violence and assault in community conflicts that portrayed exceptional women and men as having the power to use what colonial authorities described as malevolent sorcery to shapeshift—to transform their own bodies and the bodies of others into hybrid beings, animals, and natural objects. The historical archives contain descriptions of pregnancy interference, where ritual specialists were accused of shapeshifting fetuses in utero to cause miscarriage or to subvert a woman's pregnancy and cause the birth of animals or hybrid human-animals, described in the sources as a "monstrous" birth. A broader discussion of reproductive and fetal illness and transformation occurred not only in Indigenous communities but also within colonial institutions of power—the church, Inquisition and criminal courts, the *protomedicato* (colonial bureaucracy that regulated medical and public health policy and services), and the political realms from the royal audiencia authorities to the Maya *cabildo* (town government).[27]

Thus, in colonial society Mesoamerican medicine came to be associated with a wide range of medical practices and healing abilities that included barbering and midwifery skills. Furthermore, in eighteenth-century Guatemala, the majority of medical treatments necessarily relied on nonexperts such as barber-surgeons, healer-bloodletters, bonesetters, and midwives. In certain cases, then,

26. For more on the roles of Maya midwives and healers in pre-Columbian and colonial society, see Few, *Women Who Live Evil Lives*. On pre-Columbian midwives' expertise in performing embryotomies on women in labor in central Mexico, see Jaffary, *Reproduction and Its Discontents*.

27. Few, *For All of Humanity*, 104–15.

the greater goal of medical policies—here, requiring and enforcing postmortem cesareans—outweighed racial hierarchies and the exigencies of professional boundary making in official colonial medicine. The existence of sanctioned Indigenous healers in these contexts also showed the church's flexibility in counteracting or strategically co-opting Mesoamerican medical cultures.

Documenting Cesarean Operations

In seeming contradiction with the eighteenth-century proliferation of postmortem cesarean manuals throughout Spain and its colonies, the archival evidence for postmortem cesareans performed on women throughout the Iberian Atlantic world seems scattered and relatively scarce at best, though the corpus of known cases is steadily growing (and makes up part of our current research project on the rise and spread of the postmortem cesarean throughout Spain and Portugal as well as their Atlantic and Pacific colonies). For the Iberian Peninsula, based largely on research into two Spanish newspapers—the *Gazeta de Madrid* and *Memorial Literario*—Demerson has documented a total of fifty-two postmortem cesarean operations carried out between 1777 and 1806, nine of which originated in the Diocese of Granada between 1777 and 1780. From these findings Demerson concluded that only one woman in Spain requested that the operation be performed on her while she was still alive (although the priest in question denied the request). Equally important is Demerson's observation that several family members mentioned in this corpus actively resisted the mandate to perform a postmortem cesarean, and that in two cases this resistance prompted judicial authorities to intervene.[28]

We have evidence of similar reactions among the largely native and mixed-race populations of New Spain, Río de la Plata, and elsewhere: those who resisted the operation and those who fervently desired it. As in Spain, we also find several exaggerated printed accounts claiming that many of the fetuses were being found alive, sometimes several hours or even days after the mother's death. A November 1800 issue of the *Gazeta de México*, for instance, drew attention to the successful cesarean performed on María Barbosa

28. Demerson, "Cesárea *post mortem*," 224.

the day after she died, on October 16 of that year, in an adobe home that had collapsed due to flooding. The newspaper relates the miracle that even though the pregnant Barbosa had died the night prior to the operation's performance, "D. Pedro Morales and D. Joseph Rosas, practical physicians . . . with great skill extracted an animated child some sixteen hours after the fatal event, and receiving the holy baptism, it expired shortly thereafter."[29]

Likewise, in the Viceroyalty of Río de la Plata (present-day Argentina, Bolivia, Paraguay, and Uruguay), authorities claimed in December 1794 to have operated and successfully removed a living fetus from the body of a *zamba*—that is, a woman of mixed Indigenous and African heritage—who had died from a lightning strike the previous day. According to the *Mercurio Peruano*, a Lima-based newspaper that published an account of the event, they did so despite the opposition of family members. Popular resistance to the cesarean operation is perhaps most pronounced in this case, which we have included in translation in chapter 2: as the newspaper reports, the presiding mayor, Don Pedro Gregorio López, "ordered that the cesarean operation be performed despite the repugnance and formal opposition of the relatives of the deceased, and despite finding her head already fetid." The newspaper went on to report a happy ending for the incident: "The operation was performed with such blessedness that a fetus was found still alive."[30]

For colonial Latin America in general, the vast majority of postmortem cesareans uncovered by researchers to date come from the Viceroyalty of New Spain, which was Spain's largest and most important colonial possession in the Americas, established in 1535 and lasting until 1821. The first of four viceroyalties that Spain created in the Americas, it comprised what is today Mexico, Central America, Florida, much of the southwestern and central United States, and the Caribbean (then known as the Spanish West Indies, which included Cuba, Haiti, the Dominican Republic, Puerto Rico, the Virgin Islands, Jamaica, and other islands). Starting in 1565, New Spain also came to include the Spanish East Indies in Asia, made up of the Philippine Islands, the Mariana Islands, and, briefly, parts of Taiwan. Later on some parts of the Spanish Caribbean, including

29. *Gazeta de México* 10, no. 27 (1800): 209.
30. *Mercurio Peruano* 12, no. 595 (1795): 111–12.

Jamaica and the Virgin Islands, came under the control of other European powers, including the British. The archival presence of postmortem cesarean operations in the Spanish colonies, checkered as it is, stands in stark contrast to these British-controlled regions, where the goals of evangelization and salvation were less central to the colonial project. Writing about the history of pregnancy and slavery in British colonial Jamaica, for instance, Sasha Turner suggests that the cesarean operation on enslaved women (as a form of experimental medical practice), either living or dead, was either not performed or went unrecorded. She notes that while there are ample references to bleeding, purging, and smallpox inoculation on such women and their children, "there is no evidence of other experimental gynecological surgeries (like cesarean or vesico-vaginal fistula [surgery to repair tears to the vaginal wall that caused the uncontrollable leakage of urine]) performed on the bodies of enslaved women in the Caribbean."[31]

In contrast, between 1795 and 1826 there were some fourteen separate references to postmortem cesareans in New Spain in the *Gazeta de México* and four others in the *Gazeta de Guatemala*, several of which we have included in chapter 2, for the first time in English translation. Some of the references are unfortunately brief and contain little to no information on either the women or their unborn fetuses. A 1795 entry, for example, cursorily mentions that, of the 944 baptisms performed in the town of Panotlán that year, "four have achieved this happiness by benefit of the cesarean operation."[32] Of those operations, two were performed by a certain Dr. Don Urbano Antonio Díaz de las Cuevas, one by a vicar named Don Francisco Álvarez, and the last by Don Joachín Torres, a surgeon in Tlaxcala. The newspaper entry tells us no more; many of the details surrounding these operations are left to our imagination. These references are fascinating partly because they point to a significant gap in the archival record.

Building on Valle's earlier work on baptismal registers and the cesarean operation in Alta California missions, historian Anne Marie Reid has uncovered a total of twenty-four baptisms of fetuses

31. Turner, *Contested Bodies*, 136–37.
32. "Quarto han logrado esta felicidad por beneficio de la operación cesárea," *Gazeta de México*, January 1, 1795.

extracted surgically from twenty-three different women between 1779 and 1832. The women were between the ages of fifteen and forty-one; all but two were Indigenous, and most were from central and northern California.[33] Thus far, scholars have uncovered more postmortem cesareans for late eighteenth- and early nineteenth-century Spain than for the whole of colonial Latin America (though the further we conduct research on this topic, the more Latin American cases we are finding in archives, newspapers, and other records). That said, from those cases that have been unearthed by scholars, we can draw some crucial demographic information about the women who underwent the operation shortly after death. We know, for example, that most of the operations in the Americas were performed on Indigenous and mixed-race women. We find one rare reference in June 1795, from the town of Chiautla, to a Spanish woman, Brígada Ruiz, who died five months pregnant. Notice was given to the *subdelegado* (subdelegate), who "mandated the cesarean operation be performed." A live female infant was successfully extracted, and "she solemnly received the waters of baptism, and after a short while she died."[34]

The relatively sparse history and historiography on the postmortem cesarean in the Iberian Atlantic world in some ways reflects gaps and absences surrounding the operation in the archival record. But there are still millions of baptismal and death records for the whole of the Iberian Atlantic world waiting to be mined for the presence of the postmortem cesarean. With some important exceptions, most of the small number of historical studies on the topic focus on the dissemination of texts about the operation, the circulation of *bandos*, and the question of medical expertise rather than on the reality of postmortem cesarean operations. Despite the strong tradition of writing about, and circulating information on, the cesarean operation (especially as a means of baptizing unborn infants in the medieval and early modern periods), the archives contain few records of actual postmortem cesareans performed on deceased women to baptize the fetus. This is, to be sure, one of the key representational paradoxes at the heart of the colonial archives: that the operation, at least in the eighteenth and early nineteenth centuries, seems to have been performed frequently and yet (as of now) rarely appears in the extant

33. Reid, "Medics of the Soul," 101–3.
34. "Chiautla de la Sal," *Gazeta de México*, June 20, 1795.

documentation for the Iberian Atlantic world as well as other parts of medieval and early modern Europe.

As Renate Blumenfeld-Kosinski demonstrates, it was not until the early fourteenth century that postmortem cesareans began to be referenced in European medical treatises (though not yet as frequently as they would in the eighteenth century, following the 1745 publication of Cangiamila's *Sacred Embryology*). In fact, Blumenfeld-Kosinski's entire study on the cesarean operation's representation in medieval European culture is—like so many other publications on the topic—entirely conditioned by particular forms of archival absence: "The earliest testimonies of Caesarean birth do not mention midwives because there the operation appears mostly in a legal context or in works dealing with etymology. The actual performance of the operation was not of primary concern to the earliest witnesses."[35] Given this relative absence of documents discussing actual postmortem cesareans carried out on particular individuals, scholars have tended to turn to a diversity of sources through which to articulate the operation's historically specific social and cultural meanings, including literature, mythology, visual iconography, and medical, legal, and theological tracts and treatises.

How then should we understand Arrese's book in context? To what extent did it—and other texts like it—influence and inspire postmortem cesareans throughout Guatemala and elsewhere in eighteenth-century Latin America? Through the rare archival references to figures such as Chatá, mentioned at the start of this introduction, we can begin to trace the rise and spread of the postmortem cesarean as a medicoreligious practice through the global networks of Spain's and Portugal's empires, especially in colonial settings. When and where were actual postmortem cesareans documented, and how frequently were they recorded when they were performed? Chatá's death and the surgical removal and baptism of her unborn fetus were not isolated events in colonial Guatemala or elsewhere throughout the Spanish Empire. In fact, the newspaper article in which Chatá's story first appeared included equally brief references to three other women who underwent postmortem operations in the same year.

Likewise, Guatemala's criminal records describe at least one postmortem cesarean, performed in January 1797 after Maya magistrates,

35. Blumenfeld-Kosinski, *Not of Woman Born*, 7, 21.

acting as a community policing force, came across an Indigenous woman's corpse while patrolling the slope of a ravine located along the royal road near the town of Pinula. They transported the body to the capital and placed it overnight in a city government office, which functioned as a makeshift morgue for this case of suspected homicide. The next morning the surgeon Francisco Zúñiga conducted an autopsy to determine the cause of death. Among the many wounds and bruises on her body, Zúñiga documented "much bloody material" on her legs and in her vagina. These signs, along with the observed swelling of the uterus, indicated, in his opinion, that the woman had recently given birth or had died during childbirth. Zúñiga then conducted a postmortem cesarean but did not find a fetus, only "much putrefaction."[36] When taken together, these documents reveal a fascinating network of medical and religious knowledge that linked women like Chatá and the unidentified murdered woman to treatises and texts on postmortem cesarean operations in Europe, Latin America, and beyond.

Cesarean manuals continued to be published throughout the first half of the nineteenth century in various parts of the Spanish Empire. In 1805, for example, an instructional manual titled "Modo de hacer la operación cesárea después de muerta la madre" (Means to carry out the cesarean operation after the mother has died) appeared in Buenos Aires, Asunción, and elsewhere in the Viceroyalty of Río de la Plata as part of the 1804 royal decree.[37] Around the same time other texts appeared in print and circulated in the Viceroyalty of New Granada and the California missions. Although most Spanish colonies in the Americas gained independence from Spain in 1821, new works on the cesarean operation and fetal baptism continued to be published in the Philippines well into the 1860s. The publication of cesarean manuals of various kinds flourished in Spain itself. In this

36. "Sobre haverse encontrado el cadaver de una yndia," 1797, A2.2-185-3699, AGCA, fols. 3v–4v. Zúñiga's title is listed as *práctico en cirujía* (surgery practitioner). After Zúñiga finished his work, the *alcalde* (local official or mayor) turned the woman's body over to the local parish priest for immediate burial. The authorities never determined a definitive cause for the woman's death, nor does the record show that they identified her.

37. "Real Cédula sobre el modo con que se ha de executar la operación cesárea," April 13, 1804, A1-4642-39595, AGCA, fols. 16v–19v. This *cédula* was disseminated widely throughout Spain and its colonies.

way Arrese was a crucial regional actor in a much larger movement that spanned multiple centuries and continents.

Roadmap to Arrese's Work

How might present-day readers navigate Arrese's work and draw interpretations from it? Focusing first on the format, language, and content of *Physical, Canonical, Moral Principles* provides clues to the choices Arrese made to best convey key points to his envisioned readership: the ordinary people, elite, and religious of late colonial Guatemala. The detailed table of contents is followed by a short essay by the author explaining why he wrote the work and the critical importance of fetal baptism. This prologue begins by conveying the primacy of baptism—without which, according to him, "no one can attain heavenly bliss"—as a means to purification and salvation. Arrese then included a transcription of the 1785 edict enacted by Guatemala's archbishop Cayetano Francos y Monroy, mandating that baptisms be performed on miscarried fetuses and that cesarean operations be performed on any woman who dies pregnant to baptize the fetus in her womb. With this choice Arrese linked the introductory sections to the main text and underscored the critical (and legal) importance of the matter. Francos y Monroy declared excommunication, or exclusion from the Christian community and its sacraments and expulsion from the Catholic Church, as the penalty for failing to comply. Given the fragmentary nature of the sources on the postmortem cesarean, it is not yet clear whether the church excommunicated anyone in the audiencia—or the larger Viceroyalty of New Spain—for failing to perform the procedure. Yet even the threat of excommunication showed that church officials considered the procedure vital to pastoral work in this colonial setting. Having thus positioned his envisioned reader as someone obligated to learn the details of these duties and comply accordingly, Arrese structured the treatise's remaining sections as a dialogue, in which the reader poses relevant questions that the author answers.

Arrese's text is technically structured by a rhetorical device known as hypophora, which is when questioners answer their own questions. The body of the text, in its question-and-answer format, reads like a forerunner of what today we might call an FAQ: this choice allowed Arrese to pose questions that he considered important and then immediately provide short, succinct answers. Groups of questions and answers are linked together, serving the goal of explaining larger, more complicated issues. These conversations cover a wide range of topics, from the fate of children who die unbaptized to the nature of the soul and its relationship to the body, the dangers and consequences of miscarriage, the administration of the baptism, and the fate of the fetus when the woman dies, among many others. As Arrese knew, the question-and-answer format would have been familiar to literate audiences throughout New Spain, especially since so many other genres of religious texts, including catechisms and confessional manuals, were structured in this way.[38] All these types of religious texts functioned as tools of colonialism and spiritual conversion throughout the Americas. As a Catholic priest in colonial Guatemala, Arrese deliberately organized his text to achieve similar goals by instructing readers how to perform cesarean operations to administer fetal baptism.

Language itself was crucial to conveying these ideas and information. Much like other materials authored by priests and other accounts of the operation on real women's bodies (included in chapter 2 of this volume), Arrese's cesarean manual draws on a vocabulary related to reproduction in ways that warrant explanation and invite analysis by present-day readers. Words like *fetus*, for example, had meanings similar to our modern understandings of the word as well as important differences. The term *feto*, or "fetus," was used frequently in colonial-era documents to refer to a nascent being located within a female uterus, whether human or animal. The formal definition of *feto* in the eighteenth and early nineteenth centuries, according to the *Diccionario de autoridades* (Dictionary of authorities) published by the Real Academia Española, was "that which a woman, or any kind of female animal, has conceived and has in her womb."[39] But while this formal definition firmly signifies the fetus's location

---

38. A catechism is a summary of the principles of Christian religion in the form of questions and answers, used to instruct Christians, both new and old. Confessional manuals are how-to guides, in the Americas often written in both Spanish and some Indigenous language, that Catholic priests and missionaries used to properly administer the sacrament of confession to Indigenous parishioners in their own language.

39. *Diccionario de autoridades*, 39. The 1726, 1732, 1780, 1783, 1791, 1803, 1817, and 1822 editions all provide the same definition.

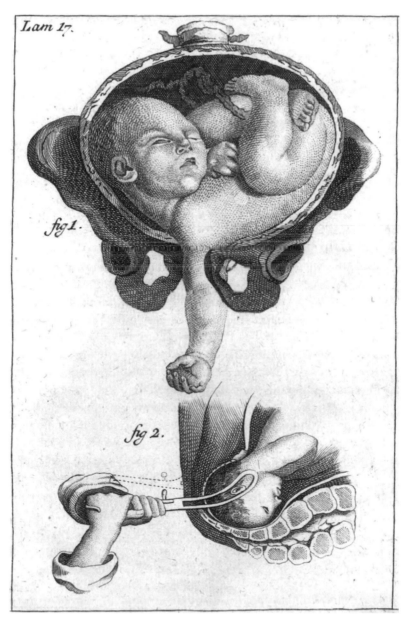

FIG. 1 *On the Birth in Which a Fetus Has an Arm Outside of the Vulva.*
From Juan de Navas, *Elementos del arte de partear* (1795), 190–91. Universidad Complutense de Madrid. Photo: HathiTrust Digital Library.

inside the uterus, newspaper articles, medical guides, and cesarean manuals such as Arrese's show the blurring of the boundary between inside and outside. A fetus could thus also be located *outside* the uterus through natural childbirth, miscarriage, or surgical extraction by a postmortem cesarean.

In addition to *feto*, the term *criatura* was also used frequently in colonial sources such as Arrese's and those in chapter 2. Today this means "child" or "infant." In the eighteenth century, however, *criatura* referred to "a child recently born, or soon after [birth], and also the fetus before being born."[40] Thus the term had the dual sense of being located within the womb and having been recently born or extracted from the womb. Sources show that inhabitants of colonial Guatemala and elsewhere used the term in this double sense as well. This ambiguity means that we cannot assume fetal location inside or outside the female body based solely on the terms *fetus* or *child*; readers of Arrese's *Physical, Canonical, Moral Principles* thus must carefully scrutinize context. We have therefore opted not to define either *feto* or *criatura* as "child," as many other scholars have done.

Advocates of the postmortem cesarean in political, legal, and religious realms employed language in other ways also worthy of mention that cannot be reduced to differences in meaning or problems of translation. In particular, these advocates strategically used certain words to heighten emotions in their efforts to garner widespread support for the procedure within colonial society. Just as our contemporary debates about conception, reproduction, and abortion utilize politically heightened language to push for certain changes in policy, so too did colonial-era writers of cesarean handbooks. Arrese and others certainly do this, deliberately referring to a developing fetus as a "child" or a pregnant woman as a "mother."

Beyond these politicized uses of language, Arrese also employs the question-and-answer structure to directly engage a series of controversial themes being debated at the time. For instance, when Arrese guides the reader through what can and cannot be used as baptismal water and under what circumstances, producing a hierarchy of sorts of appropriate materials, he gets to the very heart of what made the

---

40. *Diccionario de autoridades*, 39. The 1726, 1783, 1791, and 1803 editions provide the same definition.

sacrament's performance valid in the eyes of the Catholic Church. First, he states that the most appropriate water for baptism is what he calls "natural water, such as rain, sea, river, fountain, or well water." On the other hand, "water that has been distilled from flowers," such as rosewater—what he calls "dubious matter"—cannot be normally used. But Arrese qualified this further in the question-and-answer chain: "In case of emergency," when nothing else is available and the fetus's immortal soul is at stake, water distilled from flowers could be used for a so-called conditional baptism (that is, a baptism performed in cases where the recipient's life was in doubt and which included language linking the sacrament's validity to the fetus being alive to receive it), as could "bleach, beer, broth, or ink, as long as these liquids are not concentrated but diluted." This exchange thus reflected how religious and political officials saw baptism as central to colonial society and why unborn fetuses came to be included in the sacrament as well. The passage provides clues that can be linked to other such examples in the text to analyze how Arrese built larger arguments about life, death, and salvation. How do these representations of the waters of baptism and how it should be administered to the fetus differ between Arrese's text and the other primary sources we include in chapter 2?

Other themes that appear repeatedly in Arrese's work and those of other authors are the cultural fears and anxieties around questions of death and dying. We see these first and foremost in the ways that Arrese and other male medical doctors tried to determine whether the deceased pregnant woman was in fact dead. Arrese urges his readers to pay attention to the "usual and ordinary signs" of death, common to both men and women. He advises that death can be confirmed only "when breathing has stopped entirely, with no movement at all in her mouth, nose, stomach, and chest, [and] when no pulse can be detected in wrists, temples, or the left side of her chest." This was, in part, to assure that the cesarean operation—seen by several medics of the time as a cruel and barbaric operation *when performed on a live woman*—would not be carried out on the living, as we see in the excerpt from Alcalá y Martínez's 1753 *Dissertación médico-chirúrgica*, included in chapter 2.

Second, the division between life and death for the fetus was itself often ambiguous. Arrese disagrees that the vast majority of fetuses after the mother's death lived only a short period—either minutes within the womb or minutes or hours outside it. He refutes the "absolute beliefs of all the ancients and many moderns who are still persuaded that any fetus in a dead body lives a very short time after the death of the mother," asserting instead that "there are a great many who have survived and been extracted after one or even two days." It is worth noting that while this claim contradicts our modern medical understanding of fetal survival within the wombs of deceased women, for Arrese it appears to have reflected sincerely held beliefs. It also resembles claims made by Cangiamila, Rodríguez, and others who wrote about the cesarean operation and fetal baptism. Finally, several anxieties and confusions often arise in Arrese's work around how to determine whether the fetus was still alive after extraction. Reflecting once again the limitations of eighteenth-century medical knowledge, especially around questions of childbirth, Arrese writes, "It happens constantly that when you see a newborn child, he in no way differs from a cadaver: one sees only signs of death when in reality he is alive."

In spite of these uncertainties and erroneous medical ideas, Arrese claims to speak with expertise in the fourth section, "Concerning the Performance of the Cesarean Operation." Here he employs prose rather than the question-and-answer format to clearly detail how to conduct the operation, taking his envisioned reader step-by-step from the moment when the woman appears to be near death through testing to ensure that she has in fact died to surgically opening the womb, locating the fetus, and performing the rite of baptism. Since he wished to create a work that anyone, including readers not religiously learned or formally trained in medicine, could draw from to perform a cesarean operation and administer fetal baptism, his prose is accessible. Readers are characterized here and elsewhere as new to the topic, confused about some of the larger theological questions, curious about how to prepare a woman's body and perform the surgery, and thus in need of Arrese's expertise and guidance. While stressing throughout that priests, surgeons, and midwives should be thoroughly instructed in these practices so crucial for saving the soul of the fetus, Arrese even hoped to reach Indigenous *curanderos*, or unlicensed healers, like the barber-surgeon who operated on Chatá; ordinary people in Guatemalan society; and members of the elite. The text ends with a discussion of punishments for transgressors to ensure compliance. Arrese's text thus served not only as a tool for educating the public on an important religious ritual and a surgical procedure but also as a means to convey the duties and obligations faced by every colonial subject with regard to the Catholic Church's goal of salvation.

Finally, one of the most salient themes to draw from throughout Arrese's text is how he constructs and interprets gender. Prevailing notions of gender and ideas about women and familial honor make their way into the text at various points and are worthy of analysis on the part of readers. These ideas about gender and women are perhaps most glaringly evident in section 4, when Arrese discusses what were, according to him and to accepted knowledge (and male bias) of the day, the primary causes of "involuntary miscarriages," or stillborn births. Here Arrese places the onus of fetal care on the pregnant woman's physical *and moral* well-being as well as environmental factors. He cites, for example, as some of the root causes of women's miscarriages, "a woman's lack of good judgment"; "lack of moderation and but little care of her health during the pregnancy"; "dances, which lead to agitation" and lead her "to abandon the modesty and restraint so characteristic of her sex"; "very tight dresses"; and, among other things, "harmful breezes, noxious breaths." For present-day readers, what do Arrese's beliefs about the causes of miscarriage tell us about how he understood his own role—and those of other privileged males—in colonial society? What do Arrese's own moralistic views about women and their place in society tell us about the priest's own paternalistic desires?

The eighteenth century was a time when both religious and secular authorities in many parts of Europe and Latin America began to mandate postmortem cesareans for just-deceased pregnant women. In Guatemala, Arrese's text informed actual episodes of cesarean operations recorded in colonial archives, revealing how the debates among theologians and others transformed everyday experiences and beliefs about reproduction, life, and death, especially as they were mapped onto the female body and the unborn. According to Arrese, the purposeful or inadvertent burial of a deceased pregnant woman could amount to *fetal homicide*: "consigned to death without benefit of holy baptism, were [it] to be proven." Arrese's *Physical, Canonical, Moral Principles* thus speaks directly to the transatlantic circulation of medical and moral knowledge about female bodies, obstetrics, and embryology in Europe and the Americas.

Comparing Arrese to Other Sources

Arrese's work, however, is not the only rich example of how such knowledge was appropriated, debated, adapted, and rearticulated in specific settings across the Spanish Empire. There is certainly a lot that readers can learn about contemporary practices and beliefs by comparing Arrese's text to the primary sources that we have translated (all for the first time in English, with the exception of Sarría's treatise) and included in chapter 2. We have chosen this particular set of texts because they both resonate closely with and actively challenge some of Arrese's many conclusions. Here we identify key themes and raise questions particularly worthy of analysis while noting the different forms of these texts and the genres to which they belonged.

As readers will note, the postmortem cesarean operation and the ritual of baptizing the fetus took on different meanings in disparate contexts that ranged from densely populated urban centers to war-torn villages, provincial towns, and remote mission outposts. Moreover, discussions of these acts invoked various themes that played out differently in distinct political, social, and cultural contexts. These themes include, but are not limited to, critiques of women's morality and idealized depictions of motherhood; perceptions of the proliferation and immorality of forced miscarriage and infanticide; notions of bodily and behavioral difference based on race and class; disagreements about the appropriate forms of interaction between priests and their parishioners; and ideas about the roles of midwives, surgeons, and family members in assisting and observing childbirth, fetal extraction, and baptism.

Juxtaposing Arrese's text with the other translated sources also reveals differing perceptions of life, death, and subjectivity, both in terms of the fetus and the pregnant woman. Writers proposed various means of detecting whether the woman and the fetus were in fact alive, and they used the religiously charged terms for fetus, infant, child, boy, girl, son, and daughter to describe both unborn, often already deceased, fetuses and living offspring outside the womb. We have deliberately retained the Spanish terms used for fetus, *feto* and *criatura*, in chapter 2 to give readers a sense of their ambiguous uses. When readers encounter the terms *infant*, *child*, *boy*, or *girl*, we have respectively translated these from the Spanish *infante* or *párvulo, hijo* or *hija,* and *niño* or *niña.* Writers also valued women's lives in different ways, with Alcalá y Martínez defending his decision to operate on a living woman to extract the fetus inside her even though it risked her life (and ultimately ended it), and others insisting, like Arrese, that women must be deceased before the operation may commence. In other cases the subjectivity of the woman is largely absent from the text. Rather than depicting her as a person, she becomes little more than a cadaver on which an operation is performed to remove a fetus. The deceased pregnant woman thus serves as a conduit for the soul of the fetus to enter heaven.

When compared with Arrese's treatise, these translated texts additionally allow for a consideration of kinds of authors and their differing intentions and perspectives. Throughout their works writers conveyed information about the cesarean operation and fetal baptism with varying levels of fervor and humility, with priests often writing in a more zealous tone than others. Francisco González Laguna and Vicente Francisco de Sarria, much like Arrese, saw the publication of their works as central to the fulfillment of their spiritual duty to tend to their flock and provide salvation. Jaime Alcalá y Martínez and Ignacio Segura, along with José Flores and the medical doctors from the university in Guatemala, on the other hand, approached their work as licensed surgeons and physicians interested in the procedure itself and the provision of instruction. Segura, moreover, appropriated some of the religious zeal (and written prose) of Cangiamila, a priest, in critiquing New Spain's midwives, while Alcalá y Martínez sought to defend himself against charges of homicide after the woman on whom he operated died. Finally, the anonymous authors who penned newspaper entries likely saw themselves as reporting laudable and almost miraculous events or celebrating the application of the operation and a successful fetal baptism. Unlike priests, they were not as directly invested in its propagation.

All the known authors included in this volume were men, and the anonymous authors almost certainly were as well. In none of the texts are women presented as knowledgeable or reliable authorities, despite midwives' vast knowledge of pregnancy and childbirth and their presence at most births in this period. This is yet another way in which the subjectivity of women falls out of the records (and the very recording of history) as a result of the structures of power in colonial societies. How might this absence of women's voices and experiences shape our understanding of the project to disseminate knowledge of the cesarean operation's performance on women's bodies for the purpose of baptizing fetuses in their wombs? What perspectives do these male authors include, and what viewpoints and forms of knowledge remain silenced through their control over the production and circulation of texts?

Audience also mattered. Figures such as González Laguna and Sarría directed their texts primarily or exclusively at fellow priests, whereas Segura aimed his work specifically at midwives. In this sense Segura was the only figure to engage a primarily female readership, even if, as Jaffary argues, because of low literacy rates "it would have been accessible only to a small proportion of midwives operating in the viceroyalty."[41] In what ways, if at all, did this transform Segura's framing of the cesarean operation? Works like that of Arrese himself and the newspaper reports from Peru, Mexico, and Guatemala sought to reach much wider audiences of various kinds, but for quite different purposes. Arrese framed his work to reach even ordinary people in far-flung, remote corners of Guatemala, while others imagined themselves as providing knowledge that would be of value to a formally educated urban readership.

Alongside the questions of audience and intent, we urge readers to think seriously about a set of other questions that may guide their reading and interpretation of the texts. To what extent was the operation itself viewed, perceived, and depicted either explicitly or implicitly as a civilizing project or as part of a mission to proselytize? What can the circulation of such texts and the dissemination of ideas about the operation, pregnant women, and the baptism of fetuses inside them tell us about Spanish colonialism itself in the eighteenth and early nineteenth centuries? What can they tell us about attitudes toward women, pregnancy, childbirth, and fertility? Finally, to what degree can the case studies inform discussions about the enactment of colonial power on women's bodies through the performance of the operation? Who could become an agent or accomplice of colonial power by promoting or performing the procedure and by spreading knowledge of its outcome?

41. Jaffary, *Reproduction and Its Discontents*, 185.

Conclusion

On December 18, 1971, in the midst of Guatemala's brutal and genocidal internal Civil War (1960–96), the first of three newspaper articles from *Diario el Imparcial* appeared commemorating the one hundredth anniversary of a very different kind of event, the first cesarean operation ever to be performed in the country on a living woman. In December 1871, Dr. Eligio Baca performed the operation in Guatemala City's San Juan de Dios Hospital on a woman identified as Señora Maldonado de Savage, the wife of Great Britain's ambassador to Guatemala. Medical student José María Gallardo assisted Baca. Unlike previous cesarean operations for which we have records in Guatemala, in which surgeons and others operated on Indigenous women like Chatá under the supervision of priests, Baca carried out his work under different circumstances. No priests are mentioned in the records, and the baptism of the fetus (alive or dead)—the impetus for the cesarean operation over much of the previous century in Guatemala—appears to have played no significant role in prompting Baca's use of the procedure. Rather, Baca saw the cesarean operation as a means first to preserve de Savage's life and then, hopefully, the life of the fetus extracted from her womb. Baptism through incision was no longer the ultimate goal of the operation. Thus his decision to operate was not simply a product of the larger spiritual movement described throughout this volume but instead constituted a bold attempt to assign a new purpose to the operation in Guatemala— the survival of the pregnant woman—as part of the global shift to performing cesareans on living women that had already begun elsewhere.[42]

Baca, of course, was not the only person involved in making these decisions. De Savage herself, in fact, requested the procedure for physiological reasons. She suffered from what was described as "an abnormal organic configuration, which would not permit a normal birth," and her sister had died during childbirth in San Salvador.

42. Rigoberto Bran Azmitia, "A cien años de la primera operación cesárea," December 18, 1971, *Diario el Imparcial*, Série la Morgue, Archivo Histórico, Centro de Investigaciones Regionales de Mesoamérica (hereafter cited as AH-CIRMA), La Antigua, Guatemala. Information on de Savage's marriage to the British ambassador comes from José Díaz Durán, "Pantalones y la operación cesárea," *Diario el Imparcial*, May 7, 1976, Série la Morgue, AH-CIRMA.

Since then she had learned that the cesarean operation might enable her survival and that of the fetus. According to the article, de Savage ultimately "accepted confronting death" and asked that the operation be performed on her while she was still alive. Like Chatá, de Savage thus constitutes one of the few female patients in the sources who are depicted with a voice and with agency regarding the cesarean operation.[43]

Baca and his student Gallardo successfully removed a living fetus from de Savage's womb. Both survived, a fact that the 1971 *Diario el Imparcial* article portrayed as an example of the modernization of medicine. At the end of the procedure, Baca emphasized the importance of de Savage's life, not the fetus's, by repeating the famous statement of sixteenth-century French barber-surgeon Ambroise Paré: "I attended to her; God cured her."[44] Others at the time celebrated Baca for elevating his name to the heights of "other fortunate heroes of science." The follow-up second article published on March 25, 1972, claimed that the operation was the first of its kind to be carried out on a living woman in all of Central America, "caus[ing] a profound sensation in public opinion at that time." Baca, who had received his medical training in France, was also honored as the man who had achieved in Guatemala a surgery that up until that point "was only done—not always with success—in some countries in Europe." The newspaper additionally depicted the event as a moment of glory for the San Juan de Dios Hospital, a facility that by the 1970s, the time the articles appeared in the newspaper, had become notorious for overcrowding, misery, and lack of government funding.[45]

While *Diario el Imparcial* commemorated the first successful modern cesarean as a milestone in the history of medicine in Central America, several years later, in May 1976, it published an editorial written by Dr. José Díaz Durán, titled "Pantalones y la operación cesárea" (Pants and the cesarean operation). While Díaz Durán lauded Baca's successful cesarean operation for "providing

43. Azmitia, "Cien años."
44. Azmitia, "Cien años." Paré lived from 1510 to 1590. He was an author and barber-surgeon who attended to various members of the French royal family.
45. Azmitia, "Cien años"; Rigoberto Bran Azmitia, "'La humilde pluma' de don Rafael Pineda Mont relata la primera operación cesárea hace 100 años," *Diario el Imparcial*, March 25, 1972, Série la Morgue, AH-CIRMA.

honor and glory for our medical science," at the same time his article critiqued and ridiculed contemporary Guatemalan women. Through his writing we learn that Guatemalan physicians in the 1970s debated whether women harmed their health and experienced troubled pregnancies through their use of pantyhose, miniskirts, and pants (singling out popular-at-the-time bell-bottoms). In particular, a fellow doctor, Alfredo Carrillo Melgar, had asserted that such items of clothing harmed the fetus during pregnancy in similar ways as the women's corsets and other fashions that had constricted women's pelvises and thereby prompted an increased need for cesarean operations centuries earlier in France. This led Carrillo Melgar and Díaz Durán to call for the reform of 1970s women's behavior and dress in ways that echoed complaints that blamed women dating back to the colonial period in Guatemala.[46]

These doctors' critiques of Guatemalan women's behavior and dress illustrate the risks of misinterpreting the past, drawing facile connections between the past and present, and asserting timeless, ahistorical continuities. Complications with women's pregnancies in Guatemala in the 1770s, the 1870s, and the 1970s were far more likely to result from war, poverty, infectious disease, gross inequality, racism, sexism, everyday violence, and unequal access to health care than from women's fashion choices, moral qualities, and alleged neglect of their own health through making poorly informed decisions. Thus readers of this volume should be wary not to treat the ideas, concepts, and terms discussed throughout as timeless and unchanging phenomena. As we have seen, ideas about female bodies, pregnancy, life and death, and salvation are never fixed. The medical knowledge and religious beliefs that informed surgical interventions on the body of Chatá, for example, were radically different from those that shaped the performance of the cesarean operation on de Savage less than seventy years later in the 1870s.

Perhaps most important, historical analyses reveal that ideas about the fetus have never been stable; instead, they have shifted dramatically over time and have been shaped by concerns in earlier periods that differ from those that inform current debates. Indeed, the eighteenth-century works by Arrese and others that depict the fetus as alive, ensouled, and requiring salvation through baptism do

46. Díaz Durán, "Pantalones y la operación cesárea."

not reflect immutable, widely accepted truths within Catholic societies or even the Catholic Church itself. Instead, they were preceded by ancient legal texts and works in medieval Christendom based on precedent, in which authors neither described the fetus as alive nor considered it to be a being separate from the mother's body. As historian of science Van der Lugt explains, Roman law paid little interest to whether the fetus was ensouled. Instead, "legal personhood started with the baby's first cry; the fetus was considered part of the mother's body and only a potential life." Roman law did focus, however, on questions of inheritance. As a result, "abortion was punished not because of some 'right to life' of the fetus, but on the grounds of other civil or criminal considerations, such as poisoning or depriving someone of an heir." It was not until around 1200 that medieval legal commentators "began to treat the abortion of formed fetuses as murder."[47]

Clearly, questions of legal standing, inheritance, and salvation generated different ideas about the fetus in different historical and cultural contexts. Arrese's treatise and the other texts included in this volume thus reflect a particular moment of debate in a longer, gradual process of characterizing and recharacterizing the fetus according to shifting criteria. This process, moreover, did not move in a linear direction over time, nor did it ever lead to consensus about how the fetus should be understood. We urge readers to note that this is still the case in debates about how we perceive and depict the fetus today. Recognizing that these ideas are always locally situated and historically contingent can help us understand the complicated nature of reproductive politics in both the past and present with greater nuance. Arrese's treatise invites us to take on this challenge with the utmost attention to cultural context and historical specificity.

---

47. Van der Lugt, "Formed Fetuses and Healthy Children," in Hopwood, Flemming, and Kassell, *Reproduction*, 170.

1

Arrese's Text: *Physical, Canonical, Moral Principles . . . on the Baptism of Miscarried Fetuses and the Cesarean Operation on Women Who Die Pregnant*

TRANSLATED BY NINA M. SCOTT

Physical, Canonical, Moral
Principles
or
Commentary

On the Edict of the Most Illustrious Don Cayetano Francos y Monroy, Most Worthy Archbishop of Guatemala, Published the Twenty-Second of December in the Year 1785

On the Baptism of Miscarried Fetuses
and the Cesarean Operation on Women Who Die Pregnant

Written by the Bachelor Don Pedro Josef [José] de Arrese, Ordained Priest, Secretary to the Most Illustrious Archbishop, and Synodal Examiner for the Archbishopric

Published in Nueva Guatemala, with the Necessary Permissions, by the Widow of Don Sebastián de Arevalo

In the year 1786

Arrese—Index
Whose number indicates the folio

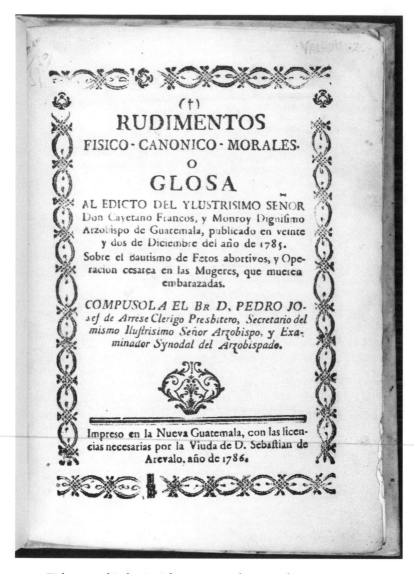

FIG. 2 Title page of Pedro José de Arrese, *Rudimentos físico, canónico, morales . . .* (1786). Photo: Wellcome Library / Wikimedia Commons. Licensed under CC BY 4.0.

Prologue

In the establishment of the holy church, Jesus Christ instituted seven sacraments, along with many other instruments, by means of which grace and the fruit of his redemption are transmitted to us.[1] But of them all, he wanted baptism to be the most essential. In this [sacrament] he provided entry to such a divine guild [of the faithful] and gave it the power to imprint a particular spiritual character on the soul, [that] without this no one can attain heavenly bliss. But at the same time that he bound salvation to it [baptism], he allowed the easiest ways to attain it [salvation]. The administration of the other sacraments is limited, even in cases of the greatest urgency, to a certain class of persons [i.e., clergy], whereas in the greatest emergencies baptism has no such limitations. The pagan, the Jew, the heretic, the excommunicated person, the man, and the woman are additional ministers of the sacrament and able to bestow it at any critical

1. The title "bachelor" before Arrese's name signifies someone who held a bachelor's degree from a university. In the original, a dedication and four permissions to publish, which reflect church and Crown oversight of the publication process, precede the index. We have omitted them. "Water distilled from flowers" refers to rosewater. The seven sacraments are baptism, Eucharist, confirmation, penance, anointing of the sick, holy orders, and matrimony.

moment in which one fears that a fellow being might die without this indispensable aid. In the same fashion he did not prescribe any age limit to receive [baptism], allowing man at all stages of his life to be an apt subject to purify himself in the restorative waters of rebirth.

This has been the plan of the Savior, who wisely oversaw the order of his designs, but, as often happens, this has come to be disrupted by human concerns. One false idea is that the human fetus does not become animated for a certain time period, and another is that the child cannot survive once the mother who carries it in her womb dies. These [ideas] have deprived heaven of many souls. Miscarriages in the first forty days of pregnancy are very common, and, as people believe that the [fetuses] then are inanimate, they are discarded, like a useless lump that does not deserve consideration. Furthermore, at least in the villages, one neither hears nor speaks of performing the cesarean operation on a pregnant woman who dies, it being improbable. Were this considered with better judgment, however, there would not be many occasions where its performance would not be considered essential. The consequences of this indifference are easily seen, and what can we say if we add those of ungodliness? There is no one who does not fear, and with good reason, that there are many miscarried fetuses who, being born in that time when no one doubts that they are endowed with a soul capable of life or of eternal death, are discarded or hidden away without first conferring on them that sacrament on which their destiny depends. In the desire to conceal shameful indiscretions with a black veil lies an even more evil act: truly cruel mothers, more bloodthirsty than tigresses or lionesses, as Ovid sang:

> This neither tigers do in their Armenian lairs,
> Nor does the lioness dare to destroy her offspring.
> But tender girls do this, though not with impunity.[2]

Such reckless abuses could do no less than put into motion all the agency of the fire housed in the breast of zealous pastors, even hurling lightning bolts that might destroy or annihilate these [very same priests]. In fact, there are various strong edicts, which have been made public by several bishops who oppose this criminal act with

---

2. The original lines are in Latin.

apostolic fortitude. Among these gentlemen we have the pleasure of counting our own most illustrious prelate, second to none in zeal and vigilance; after he was informed of the [aforementioned] disorder, he addressed this problem by dispatching an edict, in which, by means of just punishments, he instructs and obliges the women within his flock to be more careful and less ungodly with infants.[3]

This measure might well be enough of a warning against such harm, but many times we see the most elevated intentions vanish into the shadows of ignorance. A concern tends to resist what is just more than ungodliness itself, for the latter, after all, fears punishment, while the former, as it prizes itself to be walking in the paths of reason, creates, so to speak, a sanctuary out of appearances that flatters [the person] with impunity. Wishing thus to prevent this harm, a devout person who has studied and advocated on this subject asked me, as a principal act of charity and coming from a Christian heart, to create a commentary on the edict of our most illustrious archbishop, providing therein the type of admonitions that might lead to its comprehension and better observance.

It is already apparent that the purpose of this project has been only to offer a lesson to uneducated and common people. This made me accept the charge without encountering those trepidations that my inability [to compose such a commentary] has imposed on me. In a word, this enterprise is to provide in essence those topics that some authors address at length: the animation of the human fetus, the time and manner in which miscarriages should be baptized, the need for the cesarean operation on women who die pregnant and the way of performing it, [and to do so] in a plain style, suitable for common folk and with sufficient brevity so that they may understand and retain these matters in their memory.[4] This aim has reined in the pen, restricting it to what is necessary and without being able to go more fully into some points that deserved mention. At the same time I have provided in the margins an advisory notice of the inclusion of the authors who address these matters so that one who wishes to know more can satisfy his desires.

3. A prelate is a high-ranking ecclesiastical authority (such as a bishop, archbishop, etc.). The term refers here to Guatemala's archbishop, Cayetano Francos y Monroy.

4. Here Arrese refers to several authors mentioned in our introduction, including Francesco Cangiamila and Antonio José Rodríguez.

The truth is that the proposed plan can be neither more useful nor more devout, and even though there may be errors in the mode of proceeding, there is always the hope of achieving some good result. Señor Cangiamila's *Embryology* contains a fine example of this. It states that in the year 1745, when this work was being printed in Italian, it so happened that a woman, worn down by poverty, had a miscarriage. That embryo was carelessly tossed aside, in the belief that it was but a blood clot. The typesetter's wife, who was working on the printing of the book, instructed by her husband on what was to be done in such cases, picked up what had been thrown away and found, when examined, a well-formed male child alive and baptized it. He died a few minutes later, and, Señor Cangiamila being apprised of this, [he] took charge of the burial. This case demonstrates the importance of sharing in any way whatsoever such noteworthy events. But I shall be very content if my mediocre work, with the cooperation of the printer, has the desired effect and will gladly endure having my warnings be thought of as unpolished as long as they have the good fortune of being useful in some critical situation. [As Ovid said,]

Although you might come accompanied by the muses, Homer,
If you have brought nothing with you, Homer, you will be cast out.[5]
Farewell.

The Edict

We, Don Cayetano Francos y Monroy, by divine grace and the holy apostolic see archbishop of Guatemala of His Majesty's council, and so on.[6]

We wish it to be known to all faithful Christians present and resident in this land and its adjoining territories how a lamentable and criminal disorder has come to our attention [and] has inflicted no little pain in our heart, [a disorder] that has been routinely done with exceedingly criminal ignorance. The majority of common people do

---

5. The original lines are in Latin.
6. An apostolic see, under a bishop's ecclesiastical jurisdiction, is an area supposedly founded by one or more of Jesus's apostles.

it still because of a failure to baptize miscarried fetuses, even when the miscarriage might occur in the final months, during which there is no possible doubt as to their viability. This is carried to such an extreme that whenever a miscarriage occurs—without informing the priest or consulting an educated person—people do none other than bury the aborted fetus or toss it onto dung heaps without first verifying if it is alive or not. This criminal act takes place in practically all unlawful and even lawful miscarriages with such a degree of ignorance that people have not the slightest scruple in doing this. If this action, that is, the burial of many living children, consigned to death without benefit of holy baptism, were to be proven, it would result in a sizable number of homicides. The same thing occurs in the burial of pregnant mothers, even in the so-called last months, because the cesarean operation is not performed to rescue the baby once the mother's death is verified, [even though] it is mandated to do so, an expert is never consulted, and, what is most deplorable, children who should be considered alive—as has happened in several cases—are buried with their mothers under the gaze and tacit compliance of the priest and those attending the burials. The worst is that, with a priest and his assistants being present at burials, they inter the mothers alongside their children (who should be considered alive, as has happened in several cases). This act is the most frightful and serious that can occur and the most contrary to all natural, divine, and human prerogative, against which nature and reason itself protest. Thus, for our part we will do what we can to avoid such a grave sin and order that this edict be issued. To achieve this we command Maestro N., priest in this diocese, to instruct his parishioners in the obligation they have in similar cases to intervene promptly whenever there is a miscarriage—whether or not they are the issue of lawful matrimony—to aid the fetus with the water of holy baptism. Failure to do so makes them parties to the worst of crimes against God, and they shall be subject to the punishment they deserve. In the event that the mother dies before giving birth, and it is evident that the fetus is alive, they should without delay go to a physician to perform the cesarean operation without burying the mother before the extraction of the fetus is verified. All of this should be done under sentence of holy obedience; failure to perform this act will in itself result in the severest form of excommunication, a crime of which confessors will not be able to absolve them, this being reserved exclusively to

us. And so that this notice may reach everyone once it is published, we order the aforementioned cleric to affix it in the public space of his church. Executed during my official holy visit to the town of N., December 22, 1785.
Cayetano [Francos y Monroy], archbishop of Guatemala

By order of the most illustrious archbishop of Guatemala,
Manuel Llanes, Secretary of the Interior

Introduction

Question: What is the objective of this edict?

Answer: Its entire intention is to exterminate two abuses that have taken root in people's souls with piteous harm thereunto.

Q: Which abuses are these?

A: One is abandoning miscarried fetuses, either through ignorance or ungodliness, and the other, because of fear or a lack of caution, is to bury women who die pregnant, without first extracting the fetus enclosed in their womb, through one or the other action depriving so many souls of heavenly bliss.

Q: Why are they deprived of heavenly bliss?

A: Because they die without baptism, which is a condition that all souls must possess in order to be admitted to heaven.

Q: But cannot God save them without baptism?

A: According to present [ecclesiastical] ruling and customary law, faith teaches us that he will not save them.

Q: What destiny, then, will these souls have?

A: They will be eternally deprived of the sight of God and will therefore be wretched.

Q: But isn't it said that after the Day of Judgment they shall return to the world to live in a very delightful place in which they will enjoy natural glory?

A: This error, and others like it, has sown among the common people false piety and indiscreet compassion, causing great harm to children, but believe this: that those who die without baptism will not enjoy these imagined glories.

Q: So that, according to this, they will go to hell with the rest of the condemned and with the devils?

A: There are holy fathers who affirm this, but others have judged that they will be consigned to a dark and shadowy prison with no further punishment or pain than not seeing God.

Q: And which of these two positions do you think is the most correct?

A: One and the other are very probable, given their authors and their reasons, and that is enough to awaken in our hearts great compassion and a desire to succor the souls of the children, making the greatest possible attempt to ensure that they do not die without the most holy baptism.

Q: Well, now I understand the entire background of this mandate, and I hope everyone else will grasp it as well so that they may obey it, for it is just. But in order to obey it most exactly, will you not instruct me so as to remove some of my doubts?

A: You may well ask me what you wish, and, within the realm of my ability, I will happily satisfy you.

First Part
Concerning Miscarried Fetuses

Section I
What Are Miscarried Fetuses and When Should They Be Baptized?

Q: What are miscarried fetuses?

A: Miscarried fetuses are those who are born before the natural time of birth.

Q: What is the natural time for a birth?

A: At nine months, give or take a few days; any other that occurs before this period of time is a miscarriage. Nevertheless, for some purposes of the law jurisprudence chooses other definitions.

Q: And should all miscarriages be baptized?

A: Yes, all, if evident signs of death do not appear.

Q: What are the evident signs of death?

A: When the fetus is born decayed or separated into pieces.

Q: And, besides these, are there no other definite signs of death?

A: No, because if the fetus is perceived to be motionless, purplish, without breath or feeling—these are all equivocal or deceptive signs.

Q: And cannot there be some exception in terms of the time?

A: No, there cannot, because in every termination of a pregnancy that results in a miscarriage [the fetus] should be baptized, at least conditionally.[7]

Q: But is it not common knowledge that the human fetus becomes animated [i.e., biologically alive and ensouled] at forty days if it is male and at eighty or ninety if it is female?

A: It is true that this opinion has been widely known and accepted, but experimental physicians and anatomists have lessened its authority greatly, as its only foundation was a precept by Aristotle. And, in fact, what this philosopher does say is that the fetus does not move until forty days [if male] or eighty [if female], and one can see that moving is not the same as animation [of the soul].[8] But even when this was expressly taught, one should ponder Owen's maxim that in the natural sciences there is no authority that can prevail against reason and experience.[9]

Q: Well, then, is there any reason or experience that runs counter to the opinion attributed to Aristotle?

A: There are overwhelming reasons and experiences provided by experimental science to prove that the human fetus becomes animated from the moment of conception. The strength of these [reasons and experiences] is so great that they have won over a lucid and numerous following of wise men who hail from a variety of universities, among the most distinguished and learned of all of Europe, in this way garnering—intrinsically and extrinsically—the distinction of being not only probable but highly probable [proofs].

Q: The truth is that I do not understand how this precept has such probability when an opposite one is decreed by canons and laws.

A: You deceive yourself, because laws do not decide a philosophical precept but conjecture on it, prudently deferring in this matter to

7. Here in the original a footnote appears. Arrese's footnotes are mainly in Latin and refer to obscurely annotated sources. We have kept only longer Spanish-language footnotes.

8. Here Arrese refers to the argument about fetal animation, or quickening, made by the Greek philosopher and scientist Aristotle (384–322 BCE). Aristotle claimed that the development of fetal movement detectable by the pregnant woman signaled the moment at which the being inside her became human. Brind'Amour, "Quickening."

9. John Owen was an English theologian who lived from 1616 to 1683.

the judgment of the philosophers and the doctors of that era who promulgated their laws.

Q: But how is one to believe that a tiny body, as yet not perfectly formed, is enlightened by a rational soul?

A: It is not necessary for the body to be perfectly formed, as this [animation of the soul] occurs neither at forty [for males] nor for many days afterward [at eighty, for females]; it is sufficient for it to have the first rudiments of its principal limbs, something that can be observed from the first days of conception. Indeed, on the third day one can already see something like a little worm with a head; in this, as well as in the trunk, one can, with the aid of a microscope, detect the components of a human body. It seems a worm but is a man. And, if in the man's adulthood, humility counsels him to think of himself as a despicable worm, or, as David said, "*Ego sum vermis et non homo*" [I am a worm and no man], when in these straits charity, in harmony with science, commands him to recognize that he is a man and not a worm and to treat himself to a wholesome ablution of regeneration.[10]

Q: So then, according to this, one can baptize any miscarriage without misgiving?

A: Not only can one, one must. What is certain is that [when] we are at a critical juncture in which one prudently doubts if the fetus is animated or not, [then] in cases like these there is no theologian who would not affirm the obligation of baptizing it conditionally; thus, if he is a priest and does not confer baptism, he will gravely sin against justice, and if he is a layman who is not under obligation because of his occupation, he would sin against charity.

Q: And is one to understand to [do this] also with a dubious miscarriage, when one is unsure if perhaps it is an embryo or a fleshy lump or a blood clot?

A: In this case it is important to proceed with discretion. If the little growth that is born is wrapped in a whitish, soft membrane that is flexible to the touch and has the shape of an egg, one can assume that it is a fetus that should be baptized conditionally, but in this manner: put pure water into any kind of glass and have it be warm so that it will penetrate the membrane more easily, and immerse the egg in it while simultaneously saying, "If you

10. Note that this is actually Psalm 22:6 and is not attributed to David.

qualify, I baptize you, and so on." This is the baptism known as *per immerssionem* [by immersion]. Afterward take out the egg and open it very gently and carefully; if you find the fetus neither decayed nor fragmented, baptize it again conditionally, saying, "If you are not baptized and qualify, I baptize you, and so on." But if that which—

Q: Before continuing, resolve this quandary for me: I think that if you immerse the egg in the water in this way, [and] if it contains a fetus, it will be drowned and lose its life, and that cannot be permissible; does it not expose you to the risk of breaking the law?

A: Dismiss this qualm, as there is no such risk. A fetus in this state does not use his lungs, and in the same way it would exist in his mother's womb, that is, swimming in fluid without drowning, so it will sustain itself in the water without incurring any harm. Besides, even though death might occur more quickly, there should be no just fear of offense or of legal infraction, as one would but accidentally deprive it of a few instants of a life that it is doomed to lose afterward; without any doubt the need to bestow spiritual life takes precedence, for that will last throughout eternity.

Q: Well, that apprehension has been dispelled. Now explain the distinction between the different kinds of aborted fetuses of which you were speaking earlier.

A: I was going to tell you that when what emerges from the mother's womb is not an oval, whitish, and smooth shape but a shapeless mass, laced with black, bloody veins, rough and hard to the touch, or is spattered and stained with various colors, one has to deduce that it is a bloody lump that should not be baptized.

Q: In this case, then, is the miscarriage to be discarded as a dead mass?

A: It should not be discarded without opening the lump first and examining it to see if it might contain a fetus, for there are many instances of this. And let it be a general rule that whenever a woman reaches such an arduous predicament one should be especially careful with what she expels. It should be carefully scrutinized, as it often happens that a tiny fetus might be hidden within. And then, should one be found, even though it may be the size of a bee and motionless, it should be baptized conditionally. I shall tell you of one such case that appears in Señor Cangiamila's *Sacred Embryology.*

A woman was surprised by a miscarriage when she thought she was but menstruating, even though her flow was heavier than it should have been. She paid no attention to it because she did not think she had conceived. The next day she told a midwife what had occurred, who, having examined her, assured her that she had had a miscarriage. What she had expelled was immediately examined, and after twenty-four hours a live fetus was found; the latter was baptized and, having died shortly afterward, was buried in the church.

Section II
Nations Should Be Instructed in These Ideas

Q: Would it not be advisable to make these ideas common knowledge, as priests and clergy might not always be present when these situations occur?

A: The catechism of Saint Pius IV anticipated this already; it states thusly, "as there are many occasions in which it is necessary that baptism be administered by laypeople, and even more frequently by women, it is indispensable that all the faithful without distinction should be apprised of this, which is of importance to this sacrament."[11]

Q: And who should teach these things?

A: The Roman ritual tells the priests, "concerning this matter," it explains, "the parish priest should attempt that all the faithful, principally the midwives, know well and observe the manner of baptizing according to the rite of the holy church." In the proceedings of Milan, you can see the great zeal with which Saint Charles Borromeo, that great restorer of ecclesiastical discipline, embraced this obligation, as though he had understood all its essence.[12]

Q: I notice that the ritual orders the parish priest to be most careful in the instruction of the midwives; why is that?

A: Why? Well, don't you understand that by reason of their profession, many occasions to administer baptism present themselves to the midwives? You probably don't know either how far this

---

11. Saint Pius IV lived from 1499 to 1565.
12. Saint Charles Borromeo lived from 1538 to 1584.

obligation extends to the priests! So that you grasp even a bit of this, I want to cite this passage from the wise Cistercian Rodrí-guez: "Therefore all of them should know precisely what they should do so that the infant is baptized with no doubt whatso-ever and should clearly demonstrate this knowledge—that they know what to do—to the parish priest.[13] He should be absolutely certain of this, and, if he is not, he sins gravely because of his own accord he exposes infinite numbers of souls to damnation, souls that have been entrusted to him because of his calling; for this the highest theologians would charge him with the gravest sin. Possevino, in his function as priest, orders the parish priest to examine the midwives about all that is necessary to baptize well, and if they don't know and can't learn, he should not permit them to do it, and let him apprise his bishop of this."[14]

Q: And are there no other kinds of persons whom the priest should train meticulously in this teaching?

A: Yes, people who are about to be married. In the same way as he is obligated before marriage to instruct them in the mysteries of our religion should he feel that they do not know this well, so should he also transmit all matters that are conducive to adminis-tering baptism.

Q: And to what end?

A: Don't you think a woman might experience the tragedy of miscarrying when she is alone, with no one to help? Then, if the woman does not know what she should do with the fruit of her womb, the soul of the unfortunate child will perish.

Q: What? Can mothers baptize their own babies?

A: In a case of such emergency, there is no doubt that mothers or fathers can baptize their own offspring without any impediment to the holy purpose of their state of matrimony, because, as Pope John VIII says, what is done when one is pushed to the extreme is not sinful.[15]

Q: So that, according to what you say, if need be all persons can baptize?

13. "Cistercian Rodríguez" refers to Antonio José Rodríguez, who in *Nuevo aspecto* also defended experience over book knowledge.

14. Jesuit Antonio Possevino (1534–1611) was a teacher of theology and mission-ary priest.

15. John VIII was pope from 872 until his assassination in 882.

A: Yes, all persons, without exception, only one should observe the right of preference.

Q: What is this right of preference?

A: In these processes the priest has precedence over one who is not, the clergyman over the layman, the Catholic over the nonbeliever, the man over the woman, unless under the circumstances the man prefers her to anyone else because of propriety or because she has had the best instruction.

Q: Supposing then that this difficult moment can happen to anyone, will you teach me now what is necessary to administer the sacrament of baptism in the best way?

A: Yes, I will instruct you on what is necessary on the point that we are discussing. And since I have already told you what is sufficient to the subject and its administration, I will now advice you on what all need to know about the intention, matter, and form of such an indispensable sacrament

Section III
Concerning the Way That the Sacrament of Baptism Is to Be Administered

Intention

Q: With what intention should baptism be administered?

A: As the Council of Trent teaches, it should be administered with the intention of doing what the church does and Jesus Christ instituted.[16]

Remote Matter

Q: What is the material with which one should baptize?

A: The material, which is referred to as remote to the baptism, is true, natural water, such as rain, sea, river, fountain, or well water.

Q: And if one should have rosewater on hand or any other water that has been distilled from flowers, can you not baptize with these?

A: Look, these distilled waters are dubious matter that is not allowed to be used for baptism, unless it is so urgent or indisputable an

---

16. The Council of Trent (1545–63) was convened to unify the Catholic Church to counter the influence of Martin Luther and his Reformation.

emergency that one cannot obtain natural water without having the salvation of the child be endangered by delay.

Q: So that in case of emergency you can baptize with distilled waters?

A: In this case, yes. And not only with distilled water but also with bleach, beer, broth, or ink, as long as these liquids are not concentrated but diluted. But you must be informed that then the baptism is conditional only.

Q: I have heard it said that distilled waters differ in no way from rainwater, so if you can baptize with the latter at any critical moment, why not with the former?

A: There is no doubt that in the physical sense this may be very reasonable, but in the practical conferral of baptism we have to leave probabilities aside and always walk in the surest paths.

Proximate Matter

Q: Which part of the body of the person to be baptized should be bathed with water?

A: The absolution [by water] is the proximate matter that should be administered to the head, as it is the principal and noblest part of man. One should attempt to have the water touch the skin, and, as this can be somewhat difficult, owing to its lodging in scabs or thick folds, it is best to let it run freely, even over the forehead or the back.

Q: And if it so happens that only a hand or a foot of the fetus emerges, and one fears it might die before being born, can one confer baptism on the part that is visible?

A: Yes, in such a case you can conditionally baptize any body part, but if the child is born alive, conditional baptism on the head is repeated.

Q: And if what emerges is the head, how should one baptize?

A: If you know the child is alive you baptize absolutely, and after birth the baptism does not have to be repeated.

Q: It seems to me that the problem can be even more complex, and I do not want to be left with any doubts. So tell me: if no body part whatsoever of the fetus emerges, and one feels real concern that the child might die before being born, what shall be done so that the life of the soul should not be lost as well?

A: Baptize it within the womb.

Q: But wait: can one administer the sacrament to children who are still in the mother's womb?

A: What impediment could there be for it not to be administered? They are rational beings who aspire to eternal life; they can be touched directly and bathed with natural water, applying it in the way Jesus Christ prescribed, and in this way nothing is lacking to them to receive the sacrament. This is an opinion defended by many authors, both ancient and modern. And, in truth, who can believe, given the divine care of the Savior, that he would exclude infants from this unique and precise method by which all men are similarly redeemed by the price of his blood?

Q: But will you not tell me how one performs this procedure that to me seems quite impossible?

A. Those who disapprove of it base their objections on this perceived impossibility, but, so that you can see how easy it is, I will put here before you the entire instruction by a physician, [for they] are the people to whom we should give credit in this matter. Don Francisco Maurisau, or Morisó, distinguished surgeon from Paris who practiced the art of obstetrics for forty years, in a treatise that he wrote on anatomy and the birth procedure—translated from French to Spanish by Don Cristóbal González of Madrid, surgeon in birth procedures, who took responsibility for clarifying this problem—said thus, "But I reply with just one word to these sole and fundamental issues (which Roset's followers can support): that there is no occasion in which the fetus cannot be baptized while still in the mother's womb.[17] It is very easy to insert the water by means of a syringe so that the water can reach and touch any part of the fetus's body, and it would be useless to claim that the water could not be conducted there because the fetus is enveloped in membranes that would prevent this. These can be torn, should they not already be so, for the benefit of touching any part of the fetus's body. If one supposes that the internal orifice of the uterus is not sufficiently dilated and that it

17. François Mauriceau (1637–1709) was a prominent French obstetrician whose book, *Traité des maladies des femmes grosses et accouchées* (1668), was a best seller. François Rousset was a French surgeon who in 1581 published *Traitte nouveau de l'hysterotomotokie*, one of the earliest treatises dedicated to obstetrics. Rousset advocated for performing the cesarean operation on living women experiencing difficulties in labor.

will be impossible to achieve this, this objection is easily refutable, for in cases like these you must of course cease and desist, because the patient is not experiencing birth pangs; however, if she is, the uterus must be of necessity sufficiently dilated, and even if it is only open a little one could dilate it sufficiently to baptize the fetus as described before: by inserting the tip of a small syringe to bathe some part of the fetus's body with [baptismal] water." In this passage by Morisó, you have not only the description of the method by which one can administer baptism within the womb but a perfect rejoinder to any possible objection.

Q: There is no doubt that this thoroughly satisfies in the matter of the physical and material aspects of the operation, but with respect to theological issues I am still left with this doubt: in a certain discussion group in which this point was brought up, I heard one man—who seemed to be very knowledgeable—say that although it was possible to bathe the fetus [with baptismal water] while still unborn in its mother's womb, one could not confer a sacrament on it that, according to a sentence from scripture, is a kind of rebirth. In effect, how can someone be reborn who has not yet been born?

A: You have to be aware that the words *to be born* and *to be reborn* in holy scripture often signify *to conceive* and *to reconceive*. Let it suffice for now to give you this one example. When Saint Joseph left his wife, the most holy Mary, for having noticed that she gave indications of being pregnant, an angel spoke to him while he slept, saying to him, "Joseph, son of David, do not be afraid to live together with Mary, your wife, for the child who has been born in her is from the Holy Spirit" [Matt. 1:20]. See that here, with no controversy, the word used is *born* instead of *engendered*, for at that time God's child was still enclosed in the most pure womb of his Virgin Mother.[18] You also have to be aware that the term *renatus* in Saint John's Gospel gives us to understand a moral rebirth and thus what is supposed in man is also a moral rebirth. When man is engendered, he is born to sin and is reborn to grace when he is baptized.

Q: So then in the end this method of administering baptism is not problematic and can be taught and used to convince others?

18. Emphasis is in the original.

A: No less a one than Pope Benedict XIV teaches that priests should instruct the midwives in this matter and advise them to practice it, reminding them that if they confer baptism conditionally and the child should later be born alive, they should baptize conditionally a second time.[19]

Form

Q: Now give me a general rule so that I may know what conditional or absolute baptism is and when I should use each one?

A: Each sacrament has certain specific words by means of which it should be administered, which are the form [ritual] of the sacrament; they determine that action; they make it holy and are the origin of grace by virtue of having been given for this purpose by the Savior These [words] are those that the apostles received from Jesus Christ himself shortly before his glorious accension, when he said to them, "Go ye therefore and teach all nations, baptizing them in the name of the Father, and of the Son, and of the Holy Spirit" [Matt. 28:19]. Of those words, on baptizing, we are to use precisely the following: "So-and-so, I baptize you in the name of the Father and of the Son and of the Holy Spirit. Amen." When they are uttered exactly in the manner in which I have just said them to you, and without binding the desire to confer the sacrament to certain circumstances, it is called the absolute manner, but if one tries to confer the sacrament only in this or the other circumstance, it is conditional.

Q: Tell me, then, when one should use one or the other?

A: Unless there may be some prudent motive that might lead you to fear that the sacrament is exposed to invalidity, the absolute manner should be used. For example, if you are certain that the fetus you are going to baptize is rational, that it is alive, and you have natural water, there is no need for making it conditional. But if there is doubt as to its animation or its life, or the substance [with which you will baptize] is dubious, then conditionality is indispensable.

Q: And in case doubt falls back on the animation or the life of the fetus, which formula should one use?

19. Pope Benedict XIV lived from 1675 to 1758.

A: This one: "So-and-so, if you are able I baptize you in the name of the Father and of the Son and of the Holy Spirit. Amen."

Q: And if doubt falls back on the water?

A: This one: "So-and-so, if this liquid is the appropriate material to use, I baptize you in the name of the Father and of the Son and of the Holy Spirit. Amen."

Q: And the baptism that has been given under a conditional restriction, when should it be repeated conditionally, as you indicated to me in some cases?

A: When the baptism that has been conferred conditionally becomes dubious, even though circumstances might have changed, it should be repeated with this condition: "So-and-so, if you are not baptized, I baptize you in the name of the Father and of the Son and of the Holy Spirit. Amen." But if this doubt is not there, you cannot reiterate the baptism, even conditionally, without falling into grave sin, and, in the opinion of the elders, you also engage in practices unacceptable to the church.

Q: Wouldn't it be better to do away with these conditional restrictions, which uneducated people might be unable to deal with properly?

A: It would not be better—it would be very bad, because [these rules] are necessary to preserve the reverence owed this sacrament.

Q: What irreverence would be done to the sacrament if you administer it without conditional restriction?

A: A very grave one, as it would be exposed to the likelihood of it being void. This is the reason why the conditional restriction was established: for he who baptizes binds his will to the conditional restriction in such a way that if under those circumstances the sacrament cannot be valid, his intention should be not to bestow it. In this way the risk is avoided and [holy baptism] is shown just veneration.

Q: Well, so that you never fail to keep this rightful veneration, wouldn't it be more convenient always to baptize conditionally?

A: The condition cannot be bestowed on the form unless reason or prudence dictate it; otherwise, it would be a case of defiling such a holy act with levity.

Q: And is it necessary to express the conditional restriction, or is it enough to conceive it in your mind?

A: The most proper way is to express it. It is true that it was not this way in the first centuries of the church, but today it hews most closely to a decree of [Pope] Alexander III.[20]

Q: At what time should these words be uttered: when you do the absolution or beforehand or after?

A: In practice you should say them at the same time that you baptize because that is the safest way. But don't be so exigent as to have scruples should you have finished the absolution a bit earlier or later than the form, because this extent of diligence is not required.

Section IV
Concerning the Causes of a Miscarriage and Its Penalties

Q. Is there no way to avoid miscarriages? For, in truth, it is one of the greatest misfortunes to which humankind is exposed.

A: There are many ways, but not all are avoidable because not all are controlled by the will of the mothers.

Q: Which ways are not controlled by the will of the mothers?

A: Those that are due to illness and to unpardonable or unforeseen situations such as a fall, a fright, [or] mistreatment by an enraged or brutal husband, although those that are caused by this latter evil could be prevented if such extremely bad husbands were to endure the punishment imposed by our laws. I assure you that when I consider such irrational cruelty, I think of these words from Genesis [9:5]: "And for your lifeblood I will surely demand an accounting," just as though God were saying this to the unhappy infants, assuring them of vengeance that he will mete out to these inhuman men who deserve only to be compared to beasts.[21]

Q: What are voluntary miscarriages?

A: Miscarriages can be either voluntary in their cause or voluntary in themselves. The voluntary ones in cause are those that you neither seek out nor want, but things are done that can

20. Alexander III was pope from 1159 until his death in 1181.
21. The original verse is in Latin. Note that Arrese's citation is partial; the complete verse reads, "And for your lifeblood I will surely demand an accounting. I will demand an accounting from every animal. And from each human being, too, I will demand an accounting for the life of another human being" (New International Bible).

be foreseen, which can follow one after the other and are not avoided.

Q: And what things are instrumental in causing the miscarriage?

A: 1. A woman's lack of good judgment, such as beginning a journey or carrying heavy loads. 2. Drink or food made of harmful things, which the pregnant women's own corrupted taste incites them to consume. 3. Lack of moderation and but little care of her health during the pregnancy. 4. Dances, which lead to agitation, like contra dances, in which a pregnant woman, aside from the excitement that certainly causes her to abandon the modesty and restraint so characteristic of her sex, exposes herself to the misfortune of miscarrying. 5. Very tight dresses. 6. Harmful breezes, noxious breaths, and the smell of snuffed candles. 7. Fasting and unwise penances.

Q: So pregnant women are not obliged to observe laws of fasting?

A: No, they are not, because in that state they need more food for the nutrition of the fetus, who, in a weakened state, might come to a bad end.

Q: And are they, for the same reason, also excused from abstinence from meat?

A: Quitanadueñas, after having consulted with a distinguished physician about this, affirms that women who are neither country folk nor robust are excused from this part of the precept.[22] But, speaking frankly, these and other moral opinions written in Europe and based on physical and experimental reasons are not generally adaptable to our countries because the reasons themselves as well as our climates are so different.[23] Over here being a woman from the country does not mean that she is robust, and one finds perhaps as much frailty and delicate health in the country as in the cities. Besides that, the women who live in the

---

22. Antonio de Quintana Dueñas (1599–1651) was a theologian born in Cáceres, Spain, who penned several notable hagiographies and moral-canonical works.

23. During the colonial period natural philosophers and others on both sides of the Atlantic debated whether American climates varied fundamentally from European ones and whether these differences had consequences for the environment and for the health and physical constitution of inhabitants. Numerous Europe-based scholars suggested that American environments and climates resulted in inferior flora and fauna and the degeneration and poor health of human populations. Americas-based scholars often countered these ideas, arguing that such climates and environments acted favorably on various forms of life.

country, and I maintain also those in the villages, suffer from a
great scarcity of Lenten foods; to resolve this matter it is necessary to weigh the strength of these poor women on the scales of
judiciousness, allowing ourselves to be governed by true zeal and
not by that which Saint Ambrose described to us in these golden
words: "There are some among us who fear God, but it is a fear
that is not in accord with knowledge; these people set down rules
that are harder than the human condition can bear.[24] It seems to
them that the fear of God consists purely in obeying doctrine,
and all they do is demand an act of virtue, but their ignorance lies
in the fact that they have no compassion for [a person's] nature,
nor do they consider that possibility."[25] Because of the previous,
the most appropriate action for women who find themselves in
such an arduous state is to consult with their priests, who would
know how best to advise them. Those for whom distance might
prevent them from complying with this task should gauge their
own strength, and, in case of reasonable doubt, let them eat meat,
for there is a great deal at stake, and in such circumstances nature
should be the determining factor.

Q: Will it be sinful for pregnant women to carry out these acts that
one might prudently fear will lead to a miscarriage?

A: If ignorance or error cannot excuse them there is no doubt that
they sin gravely, for [here] it is the desire causally to have a
miscarriage when what will happen can be foreseen and [it is] not
avoided.

Q: Does this mean as well that a pregnant woman who is ill
should avoid taking her medicines if these could bring about a
miscarriage?

A: In order to answer you we must first distinguish among medicines. There are some that can be harmful to the fetus, but their
effect is not clear. There are others that, when you consider their
different qualities, may be useful for the mother but at the same
time harmful to the fetus. And, finally, there are others that by
their nature lead directly to causing a miscarriage, and if they are

24. "Lenten foods" refers to the food items that may be consumed during Lent,
which in the Roman Catholic tradition lasts from Ash Wednesday to Holy Saturday,
a total of forty-six days. Lent includes the practice of fasting, the self-denial of certain
foods, to mimic Christ's sacrifice and forty-day journey into the desert.

25. Saint Ambrose lived from circa 340 to 397.

useful to the mother, it is by accident. These last ones may never be used without falling into sin, but the mother may use the other two kinds if she is in a very urgent and desperate state, but always with the good and sole intention of helping the mother.

Q: And does canonic law impose some kind of punishment for involuntary miscarriages, or only for those that are voluntary in their cause?

A: In the present doctrine of the Latin church there is none. In the old church they imposed the equivalent of the penances [a time period] of three Lents [i.e., 120 days] on the mother, and even now the Greek church, too, institutes some penances.

Q: And what per se are voluntary miscarriages?

A: They are those that are attempted or sought, for which reason potions are imbibed or other perverse means are used.

Q: But what motive can so blind a mother (and I do not wish to speak of others) to cause her to fall into such spiritual ruin?

A: There can be a variety of causes, and one of them is personal gain, as happened with the case that was cited by that precept from the digest, which tells of a woman who was bribed by secondary heirs and who aborted but, according to that same precept, paid for her crime by death. But, to tell the truth, the greatest motive is the desire to conserve the luster of honor, after having fouled herself in the filthy sewer of incontinence.

Q: But in this case it seems that they are not guilty, because honor is a very fine jewel, and shouldn't all of us take care of it?

A: What you are saying is a scandalous proposition and forbidden by the church. At no time and under no pretext can an abortion be attempted directly because it is an act that is evil by its very nature.

Q: Well, if this is such an enormous sin the church can do no less than punish it severely. Tell me what the punishment for it is?

A: On this point the church's doctrine has not always been the same. The Synod of Elvira, convened in 305 CE by nineteen Spanish bishops during the reign of Pope Saint Marcellus [d. 309], denied them communion even in the hour of their death—that is, the Eucharist, but not the absolution of their sins, as some have

interpreted this.[26] The Synod of Ancyra [314 CE], the Council
of Nicaea [325 CE], and the Council of Agde [506 CE] mitigated
this harshness somewhat, reducing the punishment to a certain
span of penance. After that Pope Sixtus V imposed the severest
form of excommunication, *ipso facto incurrenda* [at the moment
it happens], which was reserved for the apostolic see, on all those
who attempted or aided in the abortion, even though the fetus
might not be alive.[27] And if the delinquent was a priest, he was
deprived of all privileges, offices, and status obtained or to be
obtained and, so debased, was handed over to the secular arm
of the law. But later on Pope Gregory XIV made this decree of
Sixtus V more moderate, reducing it to the terms of common law
in the event the fetus was not alive; if it were already a rational
being, then the terms of the Sixtine decree were left intact, taking
out the reservation of the sin and its censure from the Holy See
and reserving it for the bishop.[28]

Q: And does he who causes the abortion engage in practices unacceptable to the church?

A: If the fetus is animated, he certainly does, but if animation
is doubtful it is disputed among the doctors [of the church].
Givalino, who, according to Pope Benedict XIV, is the author who
has written with the greatest exactness about the subject of practices unacceptable to the church, affirms that it does not [fall into
this category].[29]

---

26. A synod is a governing council within a church charged with making decisions
on issues of doctrine, application, or administration. The Synod of Elvira took place in
Granada, Spain, which was previously known as Elvira.

27. Pope Sixtus V lived from 1521 to 1590.

28. Pope Gregory XIV lived from 1535 to 1591.

29. This refers to a Spanish Jesuit named Joseph Gibalino who authored *Teologia
Moral.*

Second Part
Concerning the Cesarean Operation

Section I
Concerning the Nature of a Cesarean Operation and Its Usefulness.

Q: What does "cesarean operation" mean?

A: It is a diligent invention of piety, by means of which one benefits that child who has the misfortune to have his mother die before she gives birth to him.

Q: And how does it benefit him?

A: By cutting open the stomach of the deceased woman in order to take him out of the womb alive, for which reason the term *cesarean* is used for this operation. It is derived from the Latin word *cassum*, which means "wounded [or cut]." Children who were extracted in this way were called *cesons* or *caesars*, as happened with Scipio Africanus, from whom, according to some, this name was passed on to Roman emperors and became a common term, much as with *pharaoh* among the kings of Egypt.[30]

Q: My goodness, is the cesarean operation that ancient?

A: You will find this practice authorized in Rome at least as far back as the times of Numa.[31] The Roman ritual also prescribes it and commands that until this is done the mother may not be buried, attempting in this way that the sacrament of baptism be administered to the infant.

Q: Few times will such a holy end be achieved, because, tell me: is it not natural that when the mother is dead the child will die as well?

A: Believe me, this false belief has greatly swelled the population in limbo. But even if this [procedure] was successful in finding a live fetus only a few times, it is better to perform some or many unsuccessful operations rather than lose a single child by not attempting it at all.

---

30. Publius Cornelius Scipio Africanus Major (236–184 BCE) was a Roman official during the Second Punic War.

31. Numa Pompilius (r. 715–673 BCE) was the second king of Rome and the founder of the Roman religion. For more on Numa, see the introduction.

Q: I don't understand: how can a child remain alive without respiration or food? Wouldn't one or the other be lacking once the mother is dead?

A: I have already told you that the fetus in a mother's womb does not breathe, nor would he as long as he is enveloped by the placenta. He is not in need of food either, because it is certain that he partakes of some of this same liquid in which he is swimming by mouth, and he cannot be deprived of this sustenance suddenly.[32]

Q: What reasons do you have to state this?

A: Medicine offers you many, but why do you want more proof than experience itself? There are uncounted thousands of children who have been extracted alive from the womb after a mother's death, many of whom have served church and state very usefully. Saint Raymond; Saint Lambert, bishop; Pope Gregory XIV; Don Sancho Garcés, king of Sobrarbe and Aragón; and others can serve as exemplary models.[33] But even if it had no other advantage than that of the conferral of baptism, one should regard the cesarean operation as one of the most interesting acts of Christian charity.

Q: Should it be done when the woman dies because of being injured by a strike of lightning or a headlong fall or other such calamity, which persuades one to think that the fetus has also been damaged?

A: By whatever means the woman dies, the operation should not be omitted, because in every case experience has shown us that this practice is extremely useful.

Q: So it should be performed at any time of pregnancy?

A: Yes, for in all cases one has been able to aid the fetus by the wholesome waters of baptism.

Q: And is it necessary to perform it after the pregnant woman dies?

A: After you believe she is dead, according to the usual and ordinary signs, but by some act of negligence or other cause it has been delayed several hours or even days, the operation should not be

32. Arrese and his contemporaries possessed a limited understanding of how, and how long, fetuses survived in the womb. Their ideas contradict modern medical knowledge. The woman's death would deprive the fetus of the oxygen that normally passes through blood vessels in the umbilical cord, quickly resulting in fetal death.

33. Saint Raymond here refers to Saint Raymond Nonnatus (d. 1240), patron saint of pregnant women and midwives, who was extracted from his deceased mother's womb; Saint Lambert died in 700; and Don Sancho Garcés died in 1035.

omitted because of this, for there is always the hope of a happy event. There was a case of a woman, exhumed a day after being buried with the intention of taking out the fetus; good fortune prevailed, and the fetus was found to be alive and was baptized. Verily, these are some examples by which nature thrusts our ignorance in our faces and teaches us to be more aware.

Section II
Concerning the Obligation People Have to Advise the Priests When a Pregnant Woman Is in Danger of Dying

Q: I cannot help but be convinced that there is a very serious obligation to be alert in these cases so that the cesarean operation is not omitted, thereby freeing many souls, which this precept embraces, from eternal damnation.

A: Parents, husband, people close to the dead woman, and her servants: these are the persons who should be the most vigilant that an act of such importance be neither omitted nor delayed.

Q: Well stated, but I'm afraid that many times the parents or relatives themselves, paralyzed by grief or other human motives, might not request it. Who then should assume the responsibility?

A: Any neighbor or stranger. This is a law of charity to which all men are bound. If a fellow human being is in a state of extreme necessity, no one is excused from coming to his aid, and to let oneself be swayed by other principles is to be found wanting in not only Christian matters but rational matters. He who receives word of the risk to the unfortunate infant should immediately communicate this to his parish priest so that he can provide the proper assistance.

Q: But if the common people don't understand the essence of this obligation and let themselves be carried along by that indifference with which they usually regard the misfortunes of others, and their silence victimizes many souls, what solution can there be?

A: The ultimate solution is the zeal of a good priest. He must not only instruct his parishioners on such important points but for his part should be particularly careful and attentive to become informed about sick women who are pregnant in order to be on the lookout and in specific cases take such measures as to secure the benefit of the soul God has entrusted to him.

Q: And what will the priest do if the parents of the dying woman and other interested parties oppose the operation?

A: Mussart's *Manual de Parrocos* [Manual for parish priests] will give you the answer, which is much observed in practice and is approved by the best theologians.[34] It states thus, "Once the mother is dead, but the fetus may still be alive, the responsibility and the request for the operation fundamentally belongs to the father, the servants, the relatives, and by the practice of charity to all others who are present. But when no other will do it, it is up to you, priest, because of a particular motive. For that reason, should it be necessary to avail yourself of the authority of the magistrate or to threaten to inform the bishop, it is your job to exert pressure in any way at all and take all these steps with witnesses so that it is evident that you have exercised your ministry."

This is what the manual advises; but you have to know still more, and that is, even though intelligent persons and experts in some case disapprove of the operation, judging that the fetus is already dead, their opinion should not hinder the performance thereof. In this matter even the greatest experts often fall prey to a thousand deceptions, while reason and experience are on the side of the fetus. It happens constantly that when you see a newborn child, he in no way differs from a cadaver: one sees only signs of death when in reality he is alive. Who is to say, when the eyes are deceived by so much evidence to the contrary, rendering all observations questionable and therefore less accurate, that he [the fetus] has not fallen into an unconscious state that could be masking all vital signs that show he is alive? In proof of this Señor Cangiamila cites a critical case that happened to him in which he refused to adhere to appearances and to the opinions of an experienced physician and of a midwife, insisting that the operation be performed, and, in truth, the success thereof increased the reputation of the wisdom of this zealous churchman.

Q: Well, that part is all fine, but what happens if the pregnancy is one of those reprehensible ones, where she who harbors it in her innards is hardly aware of it; what solution is there then?

34. This likely refers to the *Manuale Parochorum* by the Jesuit Charles Musart (1582–1653).

A: This is a case that can happen very frequently, but the clergy know well how to remedy it.

Q: Will you not tell me what it is?

A: Yes, I will tell you. Whenever a priest or other clergyman confesses a woman who is ill but unmarried and hears of some actions or false steps from which the pregnancy might stem, he should question her diligently to see if she is in effect pregnant or not; in the event that she is indeed pregnant, he must oblige her to reveal this outside confession.

Q: Why does he have to oblige her to do this?

A: So that in the event that she dies, the confessor can, without hindrance and very quickly after being so notified, proceed to bestow baptism on that child.

Q: And if she does not agree to all this because she wishes to preserve her honor and that of her family?

A: These female idolaters of honor would do well, in deference to this idol [of honor], to offer up that unfortunate passion that got them into such bitter conflicts and not to desire, at the cost of their souls and those of their children, to appear unsoiled after having immersed themselves in black waters. Look, the confessor should assure one of these women that in the event that she does not die, he will guard her secret with all the rigor that natural law demands, and if the proximity of death forces him to reveal it, he will do so only to those persons who of need must agree to the operation, advising them of the law that obliges them to bury this information in the very depths of silence. And if none of this is enough to convince her of such a severe obligation, he shall uncompromisingly deny her absolution, as someone who is at variance with and unworthy of such a sublime gift.

Section III
Concerning Those Who Are Charged with Performing the Cesarean Operation

Q: In the event of having to perform the cesarean operation, who are the ones who should do it?

A: Surgeons, barbers, and midwives, and, lacking these, anyone else who has had training or possesses the skill.

Q: And the surgeon is obliged in conscience to perform it any time he deems fit to do so?

A: He is, without a doubt, so obliged and will mortally sin not only when he excuses himself when called but also when, receiving word of the emergency, he refrains from volunteering to do so in order to help.

Q: And if the surgeon refuses because the family is poor, and he justly fears he will not be paid for his work, will he sin as well?

A: Yes, he will, and when there is a man of such lack of charity that he would, for this reason, excuse himself, the priest should offer to pay him, and if this is not enough, [the priest should go] to the secular judge to compel him to cooperate and to make him comply with his obligation.

Q: Would it not be convenient to have a person capable of rendering this assistance in every town?

A: It would be extremely convenient and is a most worthy task for a good priest who desires the salvation of his sheep and the completeness of his ministry. In fact, in places where there is no surgeon, the priest should attempt to have the barber or the midwife or any other skilled person learn to do the operation. In this way he would not only be doing his job but he would avoid difficult situations that might prove to be most bitter for him.

Q: What kind of situation could this be?

A: The priest might find himself under the obligation of performing this operation himself.

Q: I assure you that what you have told me has filled me with horror: could the hands of a priest be employed in such a bloody procedure?

A: Do not let yourself be concerned by fastidiousness or scruples; it is understood that a priest's hands can not only be employed in making the incision but will be gloriously put to work in an act worthy of the charity and zeal that justly inflame a priestly heart.

Q: But the risk of practices unacceptable to the church? Indecency? And possibly some danger a fragile conscience might encounter?

A: This is what David said: "There they trembled with fear, though there was no reason for this fear." Believe me: there is no risk of engaging in practices unacceptable to the church or of indecency, and, if perhaps one fears a danger of sinning, one should proceed benevolently. And in order to banish these fears, which can be very harmful, I will respond one by one to your misgivings.

The first is that there is no risk of engaging in practices unacceptable to the church. Should they occur, they are the result either of a crime or of that defect called leniency. [In this case] it is not the result of a crime, because the priest cuts into a body he believes, with moral certainty, to be dead—which is all that is needed to consider it a guiltless and prudent act and therefore not subject to punishment. No [sin or crime] is incurred by the defect called leniency; even if a death results from the operation, it happened in a just manner, as occurs with God and his ministers. But if a possible criminal act happens, it is appropriate and necessary to investigate the death; this is not the case when [the death of the mother] occurs as the result of a virtuous act, carried out according to the rules of prudence, and still less when natural or divine law narrows the exercise of a virtuous act, such as the cesarean operation. Do you think that the holy church would prohibit the carrying out of more noble and strong laws by imposing such severe punishment? You are mistaken, as this would be an unjust law and very removed from that spirit of goodness and uprightness with which such a devout mother governs us.

Second, there is no impropriety, for this could result only either from the priest performing the surgical arts in a way improper to his state or from a state of nudity, which one presumes of the cadaver, and one and the other are no more than false specters of easily frightened imaginations. When the priest does it, he is not performing surgery, for the object of [surgery] is not a dead body, but even when he performs it, he is compelled by necessity and does a work of the highest virtue, one we might call sovereign alchemy, which would purge the act of all impurity and convert it into the finest gold. Nudity does not reach a state of indecency because only the circumference of the womb is uncovered, as it is the [body] part that receives the incision and to which the entire operation is limited.

Third, [a priest] must not be afraid of the possibility of committing a sin, for the option of not sinning [by not acting] is always there, but one should not be so cautious when it comes to taking a moral risk. Charity and, further, justice doubtlessly urge this whenever the circumstances imbue the case with a degree of utmost or extreme necessity. It is true that if one enters into a critical situation, arrogantly loving the danger [thereof],

he richly deserves downfall as punishment, but a pious work is
very far removed from the punishable arrogance of pride. What
better model for us than the life of Saint Conon, a Greek priest?[35]
This saint had the obligation of administering baptism, in which,
according to the rite of his church, he was to anoint almost the
entire body of the neophyte, even though she might be a woman.
Unwilling to trust himself and frightened by temptations, he
resolved to leave the ministry. Saint John the Baptist appeared
to him, disapproving of his decision and offering his help and
assistance, but the sainted man still withdrew. Then the Baptist
appeared to him anew, reprimanding him for his lack of confi-
dence. With this Christian valor heaven teaches us to disdain
risks, which are unpardonable in the exercise of priestly ministry,
even though by their very attractiveness subjects become more
to be feared; what can be said, then, if these [subjects], instead of
emitting flatteries, remove the veil of deception before men's eyes
by vileness and menace? In any case, what should be done is to
walk with upright intention, imploring divine aid that cannot but
descend copiously on such a heroic act.

Q: Supposing, then, that anyone can help children with the cesarean
operation, tell me what is the method by which it is performed?

A: To this end instructions have been written by the three most
skilled doctors who live in this capital city, by orders that they
received from President [of the Audiencia of Guatemala] Josef
Estachería, brigadier of the Royal Armed Forces, the very embod-
iment of good government, by means of which this good gen-
tleman has erected a monument on which, better than on one of
the pyramids of Memphis, his name will be eternally written.[36]
Nonetheless, to satisfy you by the brevity to which I have aspired
in this tract, I will here transcribe the method that Rodríguez
brings forth in his *Nuevo aspecto*, one that he took from the distinguished surgeon Morisó, who, as I have told you, practiced the
art of obstetrics for forty years.

35. Saint Conon likely refers to Conan, a Greek who was pope from 686 to 687.
36. Josef Estachería refers to José de Estachería, the president of the Audiencia of
Guatemala from 1783 to 1789.

Section IV
Concerning the Performance of the Cesarean Operation

When the woman is near death, one will have to have on hand all the necessary items so that everything is ready: warm water for the baptism [and] a knifelike scalpel that surgeons use and with which every priest should be supplied; should one not be available, a razor is fine and, if there is none at hand, a well-sharpened quill knife will do. One should also quickly assemble good wine, some *aguardiente*, or Agua de la Reyna.[37] Cloths and swaddling clothes for the child need to be on hand as well.

The sick woman dies, but it is necessary to make absolutely sure that she is dead. If the illness was not sudden but rather a long, drawn-out one, there is less doubt about the cause of death, having been preceded by the signs and agonies [of death], which normally occur. In these cases, when breathing has stopped entirely, with no movement at all in her mouth, nose, stomach, and chest, [and] when no pulse can be detected in wrists, temples, or the left side of her chest, one can conclude that the sick woman has died. Nevertheless, as a necessary precaution to assure oneself of death, place a glass of water on her stomach and chest to see if any movement at all may be detected; [alternately] place a delicate little feather or a bit of carded cotton at an oblique angle between her lips or her nostrils to see if there is even the smallest movement in the delicate fibers of the cotton or the feather. If death occurs suddenly, either because of apoplexy, epilepsy, loss of conscience, or something similar, it is necessary to wait a bit longer and do the previously mentioned tests with maturity and observation. For in similar cases persons attending have frequently been deceived, thinking a living person was a cadaver.[a][38]

37. Agua de la Reyna refers to tincture of rosemary.
38. Arrese includes as footnote (a) the following text:

> In accordance with the instructions for this kingdom, the procedures that should be in place for the cesarean operation on women caught unawares by sudden death are the following: those who die of apoplexy or a nervous convulsion shall be assisted by bloodletting, enemas, cupping, rubdowns [to adjust bodily humors], and poultices [from beetles, to raise blisters]. Those who collapse from some interior abscess or aneurysm or who die spurting blood from their mouth shall be comforted with wine, Agua del Carmen, or *aguardiente*; she should be warmed with a pabulum of ground or fried ginger. Women struck by lightning or suffocated by some evil stench shall be taken

If death occurred in the way [described earlier] the surest method is to wait longer, such as an hour, and observe if the body loses the warmth it had when it had just expired.[(2)39] Then, without waiting an instant longer, the operation should be performed. I maintain that in this type of [rapid] death one can wait longer than with a lengthy illness, without fearing that the fetus will die as quickly in the former case, as opposed to the latter. In the process of the latter, longer affliction of the mother, the fluids that should nourish the fetus become corrupted, weakening and sickening it, so that it is natural that these fetuses survive a shorter time after the mother dies. Instead, with the other [rapid] deaths, though they definitely take place when [the mother] dies, the offspring is robust because whatever it was that killed the mother did not have time to corrupt the quality of her humors and thus could neither affect nor corrupt those of the child, neither sickening nor weakening it. I state this, and be sure to keep it in mind so as to counter the absolute beliefs of all the ancients and many moderns who are still persuaded that any fetus in a dead body lives a very short time after the death of the mother. There are a

---

outside into cool, fresh air; let them be bled on the arm or, better still, the throat, and bring to their nostrils something with a penetrating odor, such as smelling salts (or sulfur). Boil salted water or urine around her body; immerse her legs in warm water and massage them in a downward direction. Drowned women should not be suspended by their feet but be bled from the arm to produce ten or twelve ounces of blood, though if the barber be skilled, [bleeding] from the throat is better yet. Rub her body for a good while with a dry cloth. Insert a bladder or a small tube with tobacco smoke into her lungs and give her enemas with this same smoke. Those who expire from hysteria can be helped with the same remedies as a drowned woman, except for the smoke enema; for these women use mallow, chamomile, *rada*, a soapy brush, and salt. Rubdowns should be on the arms and legs in a downward direction; you can resort to malodorous things like rubber or wool; make loud noises around her, now unpleasant, now sweet. If she can swallow, give her a few spoonfuls of lemon balm tea or of mugwort, rue, or salvia with a few drops of aromatic spirits of ammonia.

"Agua del Carmen" refers to a remedy for hysteria composed of selected herbs and spices, made for centuries by the Barefoot Carmelite Brothers. *Rada* refers to *radal*, the bark of a wild walnut, good for treating chest ailments.

39. Arrese includes as footnote (2), on folio 41 in the manuscript, the following text: "According to the instructions, in the case of hysterical women, one should postpone the cesarean section for at least forty-eight hours and even up to seventy-two, according to Cangiamila. Aside from that, while she is being examined, her death being certain or apparent—this rule is for hysterical or all other women—try to keep their wombs warm by frequent applications of warm cloths."

great many who have survived and been extracted after one or even two days, as we will demonstrate by some examples later on. Now to the operation.

Having done what we have said, it is necessary for the clergyman to make sure that the afflicted woman is truly dead, as much for himself as for all assistants and interested parties. To achieve this [certainty] several needles should be inserted between the flesh and the nails of hands and feet; if no shudder or movement is detected, let the operation begin immediately. This same advice should be heeded by anyone who operates, and the parish priest is charged to have [these operations] be performed, for, as we already said—and those whom we have cited insist on it—the parish priest is always to be present. Nevertheless, with all that: if death was accidentally swift—apoplexy, swoon, torpor, or the like or by a fall or a blow—[factors] that past experience would lead one not to doubt her death, one should begin the incision with great caution. The first cut should do no more than to slice through the outer skin. Only afterward will one go deeper to the abdominal muscles so that if the seriousness of the accident had perhaps hidden the [victim's] life signs, and she comes to because of the pain of the incisions, these, being still minor, can be easily treated if she is in fact alive; in no case could they kill her. Once in Madrid there was the case of an apoplectic woman. The previously mentioned precaution was not observed; the incision was made as though she were dead, but the pain of the incisions caused the patient to come to, only to die instantly as a result of the force of the procedure. A huge mistake and one that certainly runs counter to performing a cesarean section on a live mother!

Numerous and fine theologians and experts in canon law have been ordered that, immediately upon the death of the afflicted woman, a block be put in her mouth so that it will remain open, and there are some who go so far as to say that it be a long, curved tube that can reach into the trachea so that by this means the flow of air for the fetus's breathing may be maintained so that it will not die instantly because of a lack of air. Furthermore, they add that the midwife or another woman should make sure that air enters the uterus, pushing aside all that might impede this. All these authors rightfully take these precautions, for, according to the doctrine of ancient physicians, to whom in these matters should be deferred, it was accepted as certain that the mother's breathing was necessary for the fetus to breathe and to live; consequently, if there is a lack in the fetus's flow of air for breathing, it will die instantly. Today there is hardly a more certain point in this matter than the impossibility for the fetus to breathe while in the mother's womb, about which one can read my dissertation on respiratory movement, which is the second entry in the volume on physical, mathematical, [and] medical dissertations. But even today, if this evidence were not available, those precautions would always be futile because, without respiratory movement in the live body, there can be no resilient flow of air to the innards, just as there is none in the interior of bellows unless they are pumped. The warning concerning the uterus is even more superfluous. Neither in life nor in death can anything from an exterior environment affect the fetus by that path. With respect to this Francisco Morisó states that all these measures are useless and, if surgeons perform them, it is more to appease bystanders than because they [the surgeons] believe that any of them are necessary (bk. 2, vol. 1, p. 360).[40] Have the cadaver placed face up onto a table or a bed, inserting a pillow or something similar under the waist so as to raise the womb. The body shall be covered with a sheet from the breasts up, the same to be done from the pubic area down, leaving precisely the womb area uncovered. Entrusting the act to God so that it may be done well and cleanly, take the knife in your right hand and make the incision, starting at the end of the sternum (that is, where touch can perceive the end of the bone under the chest, in the center of the frontal ribs where the soft tissue begins) and, continuing in a straight line, passing through the umbilicus four or five finger lengths farther down.

This incision, which cuts through the part anatomists call "the white line," the muscles and connective tissues of the stomach, must be done with caution, especially by someone who has not had much practice or is not an anatomist; keeping all that in mind, he should cut down about one finger width, which is the normal width of the muscles and connective tissue. If one makes the incision where I have indicated, one encounters few blood vessels; given all that, when you open a recently deceased person, there will always be quite a bit [of blood], which will get in the way of being able to see what you are doing. For this reason it is necessary to have some linen cloths at hand to absorb it.

40. Arrese includes this reference in the original.

Underneath these cut muscles you will see the tissue—or membrane—called the peritoneum, which surrounds the intestines and all that is contained in the stomach. It is a thin membrane, scarcely the thickness of a coin, for which reason it is important to be careful while cutting it, lest one damage the intestines. You begin to sunder it up high, making a cut deep enough to be able to insert one or two fingers of the left hand into it, so as to pull it up and keep it up while cutting so as not to harm the intestines, for if you damage them the stench and possible filth would make your job very difficult. The incision will be as long as that which was done to the muscles. The intestines should be pushed aside in order to find the uterus, in whose cavity the baby is located.

In order to cut the uterine membrane, you must be even more careful than with the previous incisions. Based on the fact that it is quite soft, apply the point of the knife very carefully, and, making a not very large incision, insert two fingers of the left hand in the same way as we described with the peritoneum: to raise the membrane and guide the tip of the knife with the two fingers below it so that they may protect what is underneath. Once the uterus is open, you can see the protective covering, called the afterbirth, in which the fetus is located. You must cut into this even more carefully than the uterus, as it lies immediately below the poor fetus. Take hold of it by pinching it with the thumb and index finger of the left hand, lifting the membrane a little; there you will make the necessary incision so as to be able to insert two left fingers. With these you continue to separate the afterbirth from the small body, all the while guiding the point of the knife so that it does not touch the fetus anywhere. In this manner all the membrane will be opened, and the fetus will be exposed and visible.

Observe it to see if it is motionless or listless or with any other indication, however slight, of weakness. In all these cases the fetus should be baptized without extracting it, with only the precaution of lifting it a little out of the fluids and blood that surround it. If it is motionless, baptize it conditionally unless it is evidently dead, with indications of decomposition, gangrene, or something similar. Even if it is perceived to be motionless, touch your fingers to its little navel or umbilical cord or its chest, where the heart is; if you detect a pulse, it should be baptized unconditionally, as it is evidently alive.

Once the operation has proceeded this far, any woman of those who attend at childbirth can help with the rest. The umbilical cord should be tied off at a distance of one finger width from the baby's stomach. The ligature shall be done carefully, adjusting it in the usual manner, in the event that the infant lives, and cutting it a finger's breadth away from the ligature. Do it so that the cut is made two fingers' breadth away from the surface of the stomach, positioning the ligature in the center and equidistant. Wash it with warm wine and apply something soothing to the nose and mouth, appropriate to the weakness or sickly disposition that the fetus might exhibit, handling it with the usual care and accustomed method. If the afterbirth is torn, take note if the fetus is strong and healthy, and, if so, then there is no need to work in such a hurry. Lift it out with both hands, having another person opening and spreading the edges of the incision; once [it is] out, baptism is administered, always with warm water, after which you tie and cut the umbilical cord.

It can thus be seen that this entire operation neither requires any special ability nor poses any danger. Nevertheless, it calls for a confident person, one who can work easily and is on top of things constantly; nothing either flusters or makes him uncomfortable. If the flow of blood or other fluids conceals the opening, quickly applied linens will soak them up. If the liver or the intestines get in the way, it is extremely easy to push them to one side without fear of hurting the person, as she is already dead. If perhaps the urinary bladder, which lies in front of the uterus in the lower region, is full and for this reason obstructs things, apply a cloth that will soak up the urine and make a small incision with the tip of the knife. Ultimately the purpose of this important act is the spiritual and bodily health of the fetus. If this is achieved, the priest or any other person who might perform it will give infinite thanks to God, having well expended his care and overcome his distress, his repugnance, and any possible scruples.[(1)41]

41. Arrese includes as footnote (1), on page 47 in the manuscript, the following text:

First note: A pregnant woman's womb often holds more than one fetus, and it is therefore essential that whoever performs the operation not be satisfied with finding only one child and thus assumes that he has now nothing further to do; on the contrary, he should carefully explore the womb until he is certain that it does not harbor one or more other infants.

Section V
Concerning the Punishments That the Present Edict Imposes [Holy Obedience,
Greater Excommunication, Retention of Sin] and Whom They Include

Q: What are the punishments that this edict imposes on its transgressors?

A: There are three. The first: punishment of holy obedience; second: greater excommunication *ipso facto incurrenda*; third: retention of sin.

Q: What do these words, "punishment of holy obedience," mean?

A: You have to be apprised that in each diocese all the clergy and the laity, even though these be princes, are subordinates in spiritual matters to the bishop, who has authority there. They must render him obedience, which means to honor and revere his holy person and to bind themselves to such laws and precepts as are promulgated for the right governance of his church and the well-being of his flock. Those who deny him this obedience are subject to various punishments that are established by the canons. Once you know this you will understand the weight of the phrase *punishment of holy obedience*: the precept, then, which this expression contains, denotes not only that the intention of the prelate is to compel someone according to his conscience but that he who desecrates [the precept] sins against obedience and remains subject to all the punishments that by law concern the disobedient person.[42] For the truth is that lack of obedience is only a fault and cannot be properly termed a punishment.

Q: What punishments do papal law impose on those who are disobedient to their bishops?

A: If disobedience stems from haughtiness and a serious disdain of the law or of the prelate, it actually incurs the punishment for infamy, and if it is a case of obduracy, the punishment is increased

---

Second note: It often happens that she who is pregnant, the hour of her agony having come and compelled by the same [death] convulsions, gives birth to the child; the latter is in danger of being smothered by the night clothes if it is not promptly rescued; for this reason the midwife or another woman should frequently check the insides of the sheets so that, if this be the case, the fetus is given the help it requires. To aid the work of the midwife it would also be useful to help facilitate the egress in case the child had just begun to be born and had encountered some obstacle or difficulty.

42. Emphasis is in the original.

by degrees until it reaches greater excommunication and, if the obdurate person is a cleric, to his defrocking. But if disobedience of the law or of the precept is caused by weakness, he is punished by other, less severe penalties.

Q: Now explain to me what greater excommunication is.

A: It is a censure by means of which the church punishes those who are rebellious or obdurate, and though its primary end is the correction of the delinquent (which is why it is called a curative punishment), it is nonetheless the most feared punishment that the ecclesiastical authorities can impose. In the words of the Council of Trent, it is a spiritual sword that removes the delinquent and obdurate Christian from the communion of the faithful, severing him like an infested and gangrenous limb; it separates him from the mystical body of the church, depriving him of many spiritual and even temporal assets that are under the guidance and the jurisdiction of such a holy mother.

Q: What are the assets of which greater excommunication deprives one?

A: Just referring to them causes consternation; I only wish the faithful really understood their essence so that this curb would bring them to what is right.

1. The excommunicated person is deprived of the active and passive use of the sacraments.

2. He is denied access to those divine offices that are celebrated publicly. He may not attend processions or the highest of all the sacred functions, which is the holy sacrifice of the mass. This matter is treated with such exactness that the holy victim [the Eucharist] may not be offered if he is not first expelled from the temple, and if he hampers this by some resistance, the sacrifice [mass] should be halted and the priest leave the altar unless a canon has begun, in which case he is permitted to continue until he has partaken of the bread and the wine.

3. He has no part in the intercessory prayers, nor can public prayers be offered on his behalf, nor sacrifices, and that depository of infinite treasure that the church opens every day with such liberality to enrich its obedient and devoted children with pardons and grace is completely shut to the wretched [delinquent].

4. And if in his rebelliousness he is concerned about death, he will be denied burial in sacred ground, and his body shall be flung into godless places.

5. Aside from this, in ecclesiastical matters [excommunication] deprives him of all voluntary and contentious jurisdiction.

6. It renders him incapable of asking for and obtaining services and benefits and for the administration of those already obtained.

7. In secular life he cannot enjoy the contact and closeness that make society so pleasant, nor can one sit down at the same table with him or carry on a conversation or establish a friendship or have contacts with respect to business or contracts.

8. In legal matters he cannot be a witness, a prosecutor, a lawyer, a notary, a court clerk, much less a plaintiff or a judge; in case of attempting to get involved in these [last] two posts, he should be recused and rejected by reason of being excommunicated.

Q: And is this understood to apply to all who are excommunicated?

A: No, only those who are made public, who are called *vitandos*.[43] But do not think that the church's authorization was in favor of the excommunicant; it [the church] was impelled solely by the benefit to others of the faithful, in this way avoiding inconveniences that would follow.

Q: What do the words *ipso facto incurrenda* [at the moment it happens], which are imposed by the edict, add to the excommunication?

A: [It means] that to excommunicate the delinquent the office of a judge is not necessary, for by the very act of breaking the rule, he incurs censure.

Q: And to what end are these punishments kept?

A: In common practice they are applied to the most heinous sins so that the difficulty of appeal will suppress the insolence of committing them.

Q: So only the archbishop can absolve someone of them?

---

43. In an *excomulgado vitando*, the church permitted another to do what had been censured. The term *vitando* refers specifically to the excommunicated, who were to be avoided at all costs.

A: That is true, unless this illustrious prelate empowers another priest to do this, or some privilege intervenes on behalf of the penitent party, like the Bull of the Crusade.[44]

Q: What privilege does the Bull of the Crusade give him?

A: That the penitent person who has obtained it can be absolved in the period in which the indulgence is in effect both for these sins as for others within the bishop's jurisdiction, however often they might be committed.

Q: And whom do the punishments established by this edict include?

A: 1. All those who abandon, cast away, or bury miscarried fetuses without conferral of baptism.

   2. All those who neither attempt nor request that the cesarean operation be performed on a pregnant woman who dies by those who are responsible for the care of the cadaver, by control thereof or by domestic safekeeping.

   3. And all the priests who imprudently cooperate in burying [the woman] before attempting to extract the fetus.

Q: But doesn't it seem necessary for the fetus to show signs of life before those who fail to perform the cesarean operation incur the edict's punishments?

A: So the edict itself states, and, as it is a penal code, it cannot be amended. But I have already told you, and I will now repeat it, that even though there may not be any of these vital signs, in no case can the cesarean operation be omitted without a grave failure to obey one of the most stringent laws of charity; however, even if the vital signs are lacking, one will not incur legal punishment for failing to perform the cesarean operation. But he who might commit such impiety will be a criminal offender who will be subject to such chastisements as those with which the tribunal of a just God punishes such a criminal barbarity.

Q: And do these punishments also extend to those who order, advise, or approve excesses like these?

A: No, because these types of people are not considered covered by the penal laws, unless the laws themselves state this. Ah! And

---

44. The Bull of the Crusade refers here to a papal bull first promulgated in the eleventh century. It offered indulgences to men who fought in the Crusades against Muslims and other non-Christians.

may heaven hurl one ray of its radiance to dissipate so much darkness so that men may be convinced by their own eyes of these abuses; may the good avoid them for love of virtue, and the sinful at least refrain out of fear of punishment.

Appendix

It happens very frequently that men go to extremes: from excessive indolence they often switch to another way of acting that is impetuous. Both are bad, and actions should better be put at a stage halfway in between [these extremes], which would save them from being a vice. Until now there has been such ignorance of the cesarean operation in our countries that its name is practically unknown. We know that it has been performed very little in the capital, not because of ignorance of it among the professors but because of the negligence of interested parties. Now that we are attempting to promote it even in very remote towns, it is to be feared that some people will go beyond the limits of the intention and not only perform it on deceased women but extend it to live women as well. And it is not that this fear is without foundation, as people in the know are aware that there are theologians who defend it as licit and in some cases obligatory. It would not take much for someone who came to consider it, should he be supported by the authorities, to go ahead and execute it, thus subjecting an unfortunate woman to the bloodiest of tortures. I am fully aware that here I am deviating from my subject, but, as this cannot be discussed without such piteous results to torment one's imagination, it would be necessary for love of one's fellow man to be dead or overcome by a sort of lethargy not to undertake some charitable prevention; this is a very just motive, to be sure, which would compensate for such a troublesome warning.

It is very certain that there are authors who affirm that the cesarean operation can be performed on a living woman and that there are cases where she is by law obligated to undergo it. If we adhere to theological principles, this declaration doubtless conforms thereto, but, as its primary foundation depends on medicine, it is necessary to examine its soundness from this standpoint. Theologians require two circumstances for a pregnant woman to force herself to accept such excessive torture: one, if there is a good possibility that she will not die of the incision; and the other, that there is no other method of bestowing baptism on the fetus. So then, you see, these doctors [of the church] say that according to sound moral precepts the mother should sacrifice her temporal life for her child's spiritual life. But the case is that these conditions could never coincide except in the realm of fantasy, and thus this matter always remains within the bounds of metaphysics. The incision, which precisely is done on the woman, is by nature fatal, as Morisó demonstrates in his anatomical treatise on the body parts of a woman, which treatise is in use by the present generation. Chapter 32, and the Cistercian Rodríguez in his *Nuevo aspecto*, volume 1, proposition 13, and volume 4, supplement to the propositions 13 and 14, supplementing his arguments with a judicious and rational critique with which, having examined some of the facts by means of which people pretend to prove the innocence of the operation, [he] leaves these [facts] relegated to the realm of apocryphal tales.[45]

But even if one were to give way in this argument and acknowledge that the cesarean operation on a living woman carries little risk, to what end would one torture the unhappy woman? People say, "To confer the sacrament of baptism on the fetus." But what urgency is there to appropriate such cruel means? Let the child be baptized within his mother's womb, which is physically very easy and theologically very sure, as already explained in section 3 of the first part of this booklet, so that absent the motive one must resolve that under no circumstance is it advisable or lawful to perform the operation on a living woman. May this be sufficient to restrain some determined soul, for my intention is not to discuss this point as extensively as it requires. He who would like to inform himself about it to his satisfaction may read Morisó and Rodríguez in the places cited; he will be convinced and will reject an opposing opinion as inhuman.

BLESSING OF SAINT CHARLES BORROMEO, by means of which the priest may help a woman threatened by a miscarriage.

God come to my help, etc.[46]
Glory to the Father, etc.

---

45. Here, we have translated *paradoxa* as "proposition."
46. The blessing and prayer appear in Latin in the original.

The earth gave its fruit.

God have mercy on us and bless us; shine his countenance over us and take pity on us

So that we might know your way in the earth and in all peoples.

Let the peoples confess you, God: let all peoples confess you. Let them rejoice and let the nations exult: since you judge the peoples with equity, and you rule the people on the earth.

Let the peoples confess you, God, let all peoples confess you: the earth gave its fruit.

May God bless us, our God, may God bless us and may all the lands of the earth fear him. Glory to the Father, etc.

The earth gave its fruit.

Our Father, etc.

V: And lead us not into temptation.[47]

R: But deliver us from evil.

V: Make your handmaiden safe.

R: My God, [the handmaiden] is hoping in you.

V: Lord, be for her a tower of strength.

R: From the face of the enemy.

V: May the enemy prevail in no way against her.

R: And the son of iniquity not serve to harm her.

V: Lord, send her the help of the saint.

R: And guard her out of Zion.

V: Lord, hear my prayer.

R: And may my cry come unto you.

V: The Lord be with you.

R: And with your spirit.

LET US PRAY

Lord God, creator of all things, accept, we beg, the sacrifice of a contrite heart and the fervent desire of your female servant (insert woman's name), humbly begging for the preservation of a feeble child whom you gave her to conceive, and guard your part and sanctify (her) with the immeasurable blessing of your grace and defend

---

47. *V* and *R* refer to "versicle" and "response." A versicle is the first half of a short prayer or petition that in liturgical worship is spoken or sung by the officiant or cantor. The choir or congregation gives the response.

her from all deceit and injury of the enemy, from all adversity so [that] she may come safely into the light of present life with your helping, and may she serve you constantly with all, and at last may she deserve to attain eternal life. Through our Lord, etc. Amen.

V: The Lord be with you.
R: And with your spirit.
V: May God bless and hear us.
R: Amen.
V: Let us go forth in peace.
R: In the name of Christ.
V: Let us bless the Lord.
R: Thanks be to God.

Then he sprinkles her with holy water, saying,[48]

May the blessing of God the Father ✝ and of the Son ✝ and of the Holy Spirit ✝ descend and be always over you and over your child and remain always. Amen.

BLESSING

Of the water of Saint Ignatius Loyola, whose use is very helpful to those women who are pregnant, to aid them in felicitous births. To bless it, place in the water some reliquary of the saint or his image, even made of paper, and say,[49]

V: Our help [is] in the name of the Lord.
R: Who made heaven and earth.
V: Let the name of the Lord be blessed.
R: From now on and forever.
V: Lord, hear my prayer.
R: And let my cry come unto you.
V: The Lord be with you.
R: And with your spirit.

48. This line appears in Spanish in the original.
49. The first two sentences of this blessing appear in Spanish in the original. The rest appears in Latin, along with the two prayers that follow.

Let Us Pray.

Lord Holy Father, almighty eternal God, who, by pouring the grace of your blessing on the sick, guard your handiwork with vast piety to the calling of your name; be present kindly; and, with the intercession of the Blessed Virgin Mary and Holy Father Ignatius, raise up with your right hand your servants freed from sickness and endowed with health; strengthen with virtue; guard with might; and restore (them) with all the prosperity of your holy church, through Christ our Lord, Amen.

Blessed Lord, establish this water to be a remedy in health for humans and, through the intercession of the Blessed Virgin Mary and Holy Father Ignatius, whose relic [or] picture is immersed in it so that whoever is filled with it may receive health of body and security of spirit. Through Christ our Lord, Amen.

Let Us Pray.

Bestow, most blessed God, on this water, through the contact with the relic or the image of your holy Ignatius, the power of healing the body and spirit and driving all ills from this place and its inhabitants. In the name of the Father and the Son and the Holy Spirit, Amen.

God, who to propagate the greater glory of your name has strengthened the church militant with the new help of blessed Ignatius, grant that, with his help and by imitating [him] as we struggle on earth, we, crowned with him, might earn merit in heaven through Christ our Lord. Amen.

A. M. D. G. ["To the greater glory of God"]

2

Additional Translations from Across the Spanish Empire

Excerpt from Spain

Jaime Alcalá y Martínez, Dissertación médico-chirúrgica sobre una operación cesárea, executada en muger, y feto vivos en esta Ciudad de Valencia (*Valencia: Viuda de Conejos, 1753*), 1–10

[Although the cesarean operation is today regularly performed on living women and is considered safe, in the eighteenth century this was not so. At that time the operation was thought to lead almost certainly to the woman's death, since surgical knowledge was limited and the possibility of an infection at the site of the incision was high. Writers such as Pedro José de Arrese in Guatemala and Antonio José Rodríguez and Francesco Cangiamila in Europe therefore argued that it should never be performed on living women but rather should be reserved for those who had already died, to extract and baptize the fetus inside them. The account that follows, written by surgeon Jaime Alcalá y Martínez of Valencia, Spain, in 1753, is one of the few examples we have of a cesarean operation performed on a living woman. Alcalá y Martínez defends his decision and that of the local physician, Jaime Matheo Fuertes, and the midwife, Vicenta Iñego, to operate on María Ivañez, given their belief that she would otherwise almost certainly perish. When Ivañez subsequently died, Alcalá y Martínez blamed the outcome not on the operation itself but instead on the carelessness of those assisting in her recovery. He took credit,

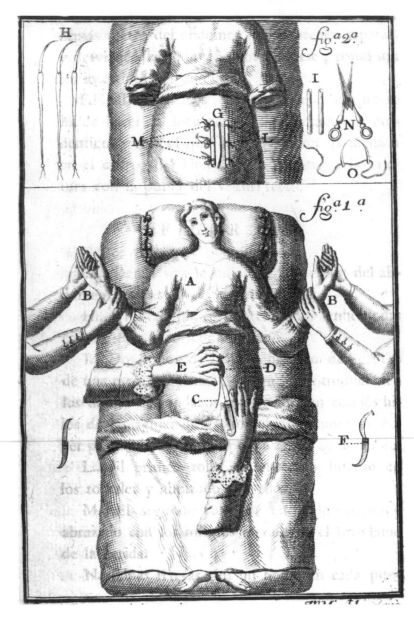

FIG. 3 *Image of Woman Undergoing a Cesarean Operation.* From José Ventura Pastor, *Preceptos generales sobre las operaciones de los partos* (1790). Universidad Complutense de Madrid. Photo: HathiTrust Digital Library.

moreover, for the newborn child's survival. In Valencia, however, residents saw the operation as barbaric and dangerous and accused him of homicide.]

Dissertation

The Holy Spirit, exhorting all to take care of a good name, *curam habe de bono nomine*, moves me to write the present dissertation to preserve my own name, which others have sought to cloud, for goals that God only knows, in light of the aforementioned operation that I carried out, in the way that I will later tell.[1]

On the twenty-sixth day of January of this year of 1753, having been summoned to attend to María Ivañez, forty years of age, I found her fatigued from a difficult birth, in which having already broken the membranes, or amniotic sac, the feto showed only its right hand. Virenia Iñego, the midwife, or *obstetriz*, who attended to the birth, saw this.[2] She was unable to find the head or any other member at all or to turn the feto around, and she joined others in calling Dr. D. Jaime Matheo Fuertes, the doctor of this city of Valencia, so that he could resolve the difficulty expressed here. He prescribed a bleeding, which was carried out later. Having been charged by the midwife with examining the birth and helping her, I found that the feto had extended its hand through the natural path, but in such a way that the head could not be found, nor any other member, so as to turn it around.[3] And even when [the fetus's] right hand was inserted back into the uterus, it would later extend [the hand] again. Because the case was such an arduous one, I applied the *speculum matricis*, but without being able to discover, even by this means, any member at all or to move it [the fetus] into another position.[4] In consequence of this I called the aforementioned physician and the midwife, the latter of whom said she no longer knew what to do, since she judged everything to be done in vain, given the great difficulty of the birth. [She judged] that the mother and feto would both die unless the manual operation was carried out, which she left

1. The original phrase, "take care of a good name," is in Latin. Here Alcalá y Martínez draws from Ecclesiasticus 41, which emphasizes preservation of one's good name.
2. *Obstetriz* is midwife in Latin.
3. Natural path refers to the birth canal, described as *vía natural* in the original.
4. *Speculum matricis* is likely some version of a speculum, an instrument used to open the cervix.

in my charge and diligence.[5] I made this same judgment myself and [concluded] that the mother and feto were necessarily threatened with death in [these] instances, due to the bad situation in which the feto found itself. And [I came to this conclusion] as well due to the substantial hemorrhaging of blood that the woman in labor suffered, which was considerable and born of the violent extension with which the uterus was found, which caused the blood vessels to extend and rupture, causing this horrible and fatal symptom. And not trusting the survival of either [the woman's or the fetus's] life in accordance with the prognoses of said doctor and midwife and heeding the sixth sentence of book 1, "For extreme illnesses, extreme remedies are most suitable," I proposed that the cesarean operation be carried out, following the system of the most knowledgeable, distinguished, and worthy-of-being-read Don Lorenzo Heister, with whom, and with the help of God, I entrusted the saving of the two lives, or at least one of them, because this is an operation that does not aim to take away life directly but rather to give life to both.[6] And in the most desperate of cases it is better, or at least less bad, to experiment with a doubtful remedy than to leave the sick condemned to a certain and inevitable death, as the acclaimed Heister has many times admonished, following the famous Hippocrates and the common [view] of the authors. It is fate, then, that the physician or surgeon is judged to be cruel and heartless, who, being suspicious of the many signs of life of the sick and having a remedy, although it might be a doubtful or not completely certain one (from which some good effect, and also life, may result), fails to carry it out, without heeding the sentence of Celsus: "Doubtful hope is better than despair of a cure."[7] And considering that the cesarean operation is nothing more than a wound penetrating the natural cavity and that from this one can usually be healed, as the observations of many of the famous classical authors confirm, and as Heister says that this operation is of no more consequence than that of a lithotomy, which is carried out and from which one is usually healed, it then follows that one can also carry out and practice the cesarean, since it is not as dangerous as trepanation in the

5. Manual operation refers to the cesarean operation.
6. The original sentence, "For extreme illnesses, extreme remedies are most suitable," is in Latin.
7. The original sentence, "Doubtful hope is better than despair of a cure," is in Latin.

animal cavity or the draining of fluids from the vital cavity through an incision in order to remove materials contained there that, if not extracted, would inevitably lead to death and that, if removed, usually [enable the patient] to live.[8] This is experienced in the most principal and dangerous cavities, so why, in similar cases, has the cesarean not been carried out?

Having heard all of this, the aforementioned Dr. D. Jaime Matheo Fuertes said that he was of the same opinion as me, since otherwise the deaths of the mother and the feto would be certain and inevitable, because of the symptoms and circumstances that accompany the woman in labor, as has been said. For this reason he decided that the aforementioned operation would be put into practice, preparing on his part some tonics, as is required in this case. The midwife, or obstetriz, said that she judged as infallible the death of both [the woman and the fetus], since the copious and continuous flow of blood that the woman in labor experienced was cause enough for her to die soon, and thus it was a pious remedy to try to give life to them, where nobody had hoped [for such a thing]. With this assumption we agreed to execute the operation at five in the afternoon, preceded by the woman in labor receiving the holy sacraments.

And, given that in rare and difficult cases it is prudent to consult and confer with knowledgeable and expert men in the field, I consulted about this [case] and all its circumstances with Sr. D. Juan Gómez, schoolteacher and subdelegate examiner of surgery for the royal *protomedicato* of the city of Valencia, who, noting all the circumstances, said that it was a very pious and just proposal [to operate], and it conformed to reason, law, and justice, and that one's conscience obligated one to carry it out, which meant that I would not fulfill my obligation if I stopped practicing the well-known operation and that I am well justified in following the doctrine and method of the most knowledgeable Heister.[9]

Everything mentioned here so far had already occurred in conformity with the sentence of Ovid, which is that one should try everything first, but the incurable incision should be made so as to not infect the healthy part: All means must be tried first, but an incurable

---

8. Lithotomy is the surgical removal of a kidney stone, bladder stone, gallstone, or similar calculi.

9. The *protomedicato* is the tribunal of the medical examiner.

wound must be cut away by the blade, lest the healthy part becomes infected.[10] With the decision of the aforementioned Sr. D. Juan Gómez, I entered into the operation, for the execution of which I provided three assistants, or ministers, practitioners, and interns of mine in said field, the names of whom were Miguel Richart, Francisco Salom, and Manuel Ruíz. And even then, before arriving at the operation, I tried to see whether I could help the patient through the use of my hands [alone], but in no way could I move the positioning of the feto. Witnessing this insurmountable difficulty, I decided to undertake the operation, warning that the mother was found to still have much strength in the midst of having been expelling large clots of blood from the natural path all day, which alone was sufficient to necessarily bring about the death of said woman. And, heeding what the famous and praiseworthy Heister warns us, which is that although great loss of blood may be observed before or after the operation, we should not let this frighten us. And, considering that this relentless flow could be corrected with the operation, I sought to explore whether the feto was alive or not, which I determined by squeezing its fingers, since it then began to move them. And, knowing that it was alive, I baptized it conditionally.[11] And with all the assistants prepared, I arranged them in the following form: the first on the right side, holding the [woman's] right hand and foot; the second on the left side, firmly taking the left hand and foot, and I gave the source of light and bandages to the third. With this arrangement I began my operation, putting my hand in between the muscles, and with the scalpel I divided the common teguments, making a longitudinal line some seven transversal inches long on the right side, [and] four transversal inches near the white line in the hypogastric region, between the pubis and the umbilical region. And I proceeded dividing the muscles of the abdomen—that is to say, the descending oblique, ascending oblique, and the transversal. Then I passed with the curved scissors [cutting] to the peritoneum, and from there to the uterus, which I also divided, and I cleaned the wound with a sponge dampened with tepid wine. But such little blood came out of there, that it [the operation] for me occurred with the same blessedness as for Miguel Doringio, who refers to a cesarean operation that he

10. The original sentence is in Latin.
11. The original term, "conditionally," is in Latin.

carried out with both the mother and feto alive, and his took place without any shedding of blood, and with very little pain, as all the assistants observed. And after the afterbirth became visible, with the feto unable to leave because it was enclosed in the uterus and blocked by the pubic bone, I decided to insert my hand through the natural path, and, taking the arm of the feto and pushing it forcefully toward its chest, I obligated it [the fetus] to leave through the aforementioned incision. After it was extracted, it began to cry, manifesting the blessedness of being removed alive and without injury, and it was a very handsome girl. It became clear that the head had been behind the pubic bone and that the umbilical cord had been wrapped around the neck three times, a most sufficient cause for her to have been strangled.

Once the afterbirth was removed, I dressed the wound, encouraging it [to heal] with tepid wine, and once I completed the gastroraphia of the corresponding separation, the operation ended so blessedly that, beyond the shedding of little blood, once concluded, not even a drop of blood was visible externally or in the natural path, this grave and mortal accident having ended up corrected.[12] And, likewise, the patient was without pain already (which she felt only very lightly in the operation) and very rested and without fatigue, saying that she was already in much repose and that she felt only some weakness, similar to what she experienced before the operation, caused by the great shedding of blood that had happened before.

With this completed I charged the aforementioned physician Don Jaime Matheo to administer some tonics and treatments and to monitor the patient's diet, because she really had emerged from the operation so blessedly that the physician and the midwife, or obstetriz, remained satisfied and very pleased.

On the next day Señor D. Jaime Matheo and I came across the patient quite improved and recovered, without pain, and, when we uncovered the wound, we found it without inflammation or any other feature. We applied to it some cloth dampened in wine spirits and then the ligature, and I ordered that the girl be taken to the church to be baptized. The following night those present found [the mother] much better and, without finding new concerns, wanted to leave. And when they went to see her [again], they found her dead,

---

12. Gastroraphia is a technique of suturing.

attributing this unintended case to the carelessness of those present to assist her, as they themselves confirmed. And this is what our divine Hippocrates expresses so much in the first of his aphorisms, section 1, near the end: the physician must not only be prepared to do what is right himself but also make the patient, the attendant, and externals cooperate.[13]

[*Translated by Adam Warren*]

Excerpts from Colonial Peru and Río de la Plata

Francisco González Laguna, El zelo sacerdotal para con los niños no-nacidos (*Lima: Imprenta de los Huérfanos, 1781*)

[*In 1780 and 1781, massive rebellions largely of Indigenous people swept across the Andean highlands of Peru and Upper Peru (present-day Bolivia), threatening to end Spanish colonial rule. This introductory passage from Francisco González Laguna's* El zelo sacerdotal para con los niños no-nacidos *tells of a particularly gruesome battle to convey the spiritual urgency for introducing and requiring the cesarean operation and fetal baptism. The author alleges that rebels in the village of San Pedro de Buenavista employed the battle tactic of not only slaughtering pregnant women but also cutting open their abdomens to remove the unborn fetuses inside them, thereby ensuring their deaths. Witnessing this, a heroic priest entered the battlefield with holy water to baptize the unborn, until he too was killed. While it is unclear whether this battle actually occurred and whether the atrocities ever took place as described, the story enabled González Laguna to reframe the cesarean operation and fetal baptism as part of an ongoing campaign against what he perceived to be barbarism among Indigenous people. In this way he embraced racist stereotypes of Indigenous people as uncivilized and inherently savage, and he rendered the operation part of priests' mission of evangelization in the Americas.*]

---

13. The quoted phrase after the colon is in Latin.

Note

We do not wish to defraud the edification and memory of a recent event announced with sufficient authenticity, in which pastoral zeal, shining and emulating that [which was] seen in the church in the first centuries, offers parish priests and presbyters in posterity a new model of apostolic fearlessness for saving the souls of the unborn children.

In the month of March of this year in the parish and village of San Pedro de Buenavista, province of Chayanta, archbishopric of Charcas, of the Viceroyalty of Buenos Aires, the rebel Indians attacked with ultimate force, numbering sevenfold against the Spanish and mestizo residents, whom the priest and most esteemed and erudite man Don Ysidro Herrera had defended in the sanctuary of his church from four or five invasions carried out since the previous September. In this last battle they had survived six days with their wives and children in the shadow of the sacred and the protection of their pastor [when], sensing that this last period of living had arrived in the midst of the overpowering and rapid outburst of the barbarians, [the priest,] dressing himself in a surplice and stole and taking the crucifix in his hands, exhorted his flock to receive death in the spirit of penitence and exhorted five priests who accompanied him (among them a brother of his named Domingo) as much as possible to watch over, as his loyal assistants, the needs of those victims. The insurgents soon descended, slitting throats and killing without restraint. Wishing to finish off even the most delicate race of those besieged, they sliced open the bellies of pregnant women and raised up their tender infants on the points of their swords like martial trophies. Horrified by this cruelty as much as he was taken by the zeal of his devout brother, Dr. D. Domingo hurled himself fearlessly into the middle of the carnage to grab and baptize the unborn infants, judging this to be the greatest need and without fearing death, and he kept pouring holy water onto their innocent blood until, by shedding his own blood, he ended his career gloriously. The four remaining priests followed his example while he was still alive and encouraged them through continuous exhortation, and the sacrilegious ire of the rebels had nothing left to destroy after 1,400 dead, who were the congregants.

[Translated by Adam Warren]

El Mercurio Peruano *12, no. 595 (1795): 111–12.*

[*Unlike in colonial Mexico and Guatemala, where news of the cesarean operation's use appeared numerous times in newspapers and gazettes at the end of the eighteenth century and the start of the nineteenth, in Peru such announcements were rare. To our knowledge this article from* El Mercurio Peruano, *Lima's leading Enlightenment newspaper, about an operation performed in 1794 is the only one of its kind. The article describes the death of a pregnant woman struck by lightning in Tucumán, a city in present-day northwestern Argentina that had formed part of Peru prior to the creation of the Viceroyalty of Río de la Plata in 1776. The article tells how ecclesiastical and government authorities insisted on and coordinated the operation despite the objections of family members. The alleged survival of the unborn fetus overnight in the deceased woman's womb, as described in the text, is medically impossible, but the narrative serves as clear propaganda for the operation's value.*]

Tucumán, January 8, 1795.

On the eighteenth day of last December, at around half past five in the afternoon, a lightning bolt killed a pregnant *zamba* in the later months of [her] pregnancy.[14] It entered her through half of her skull, exited from her right side, and ran superficially all through the rest of her body as far as her knees. With agreement from the vicar priest of this city, Don Joseph Ignacio Tames, on the following nineteenth day the presiding mayor of the city council, Don Pedro Gregorio López, ordered that the cesarean operation be performed despite the repugnance and formal opposition of the relatives of the deceased and despite finding her head already fetid. Indeed, at eleven thirty in the morning, Don Antonio Terri happily carried out the operation in the presence of the said mayor and vicar as well as other gentlemen, who came together with pleasure for it. The operation was performed with such blessedness that a feto was found still alive. It was a male, and he lasted a quarter of an hour after the baptism. There is no doubt that the criatura would have lived if the operation had been performed right after the misfortune took place, but the mourners of the

14. A *zamba* is a person of Indigenous and African parentage.

deceased kept a pernicious silence in the midst of seeing the criatura move within the belly without ceasing. This case proves no less the importance of the operation than the vigilance with which we should all oppose those peoples who are careless on a point so important for the health of the soul and of the body.

[*Translated by Adam Warren*]

Excerpts from Colonial Guatemala

"Despacho del sup[eri]or gobierno para que se haga practicar la operación cesárea," February 16, 1786, A1-6098-55547, Archivo General de Centro América, Guatemala City, fols. 1r–17v, 2r–4v

[*In conjunction with the decree mandating postmortem cesareans, audiencia president Don José de Estachería commissioned medical doctors at the University of San Carlos to write the official instructions detailing how to conduct the procedure and adapt it to local conditions, including in Indigenous communities and rural areas. In 1786 these instructions, bundled with the postmortem cesarean mandate, were sent to officials throughout Central America. Estachería intended the instructions to be used by nonmedical specialists such as priests, barber-surgeons, and midwives, as the goal was to provide "a succinct instruction, methodical and clear, of how to carry out the said [cesarean] procedure so that finally in all the provinces of [Central America] one can follow the instructions without the need for profesores [medical physicians and surgeons with university medical degrees]." The following is an extract from these instructions, concerned with telling the reader what death signs to look for on a pregnant woman's body. Such signs would enable the reader to identify the precise moment of death so that a cesarean may be immediately conducted, thus ensuring the best chance of a successful fetal baptism.*]

Precautions that must be taken [when conducting a postmortem cesarean operation on women] who die from a chronic or acute illness.

A chronic or long illness is defined as a sickness that lasts a considerable amount of time [until death], such as from dropsy, *hética*, *tipsica*, [or] diarrhea, more commonly known as *evacuaciones*.[15]

An acute illness lasts only for a short time [before death], usually either seven, eleven, or fourteen days, such as fevers associated with typhus, diphtheria, rabies, and so on.[16]

When a pregnant woman has died from some chronic illness, one sees clearly how the illness quickly becomes so serious that the sick woman becomes prostrate, weakening more each day, followed by swooning, cold sweats, and death throes; then she will lack a pulse and [no longer] breathe.

In the same manner, when a woman with an acute illness is about to die, one observes a delirium that they call *disvario*, [or] the spasmodic movement of the diaphragm; convulsions; [and] fainting spells, which are the death throes, and [then] she dies. Weakness, swooning, delirium, the spasmodic movement of the diaphragm, convulsions, cold sweats, the disappearance of the pulse, death throes, and so on are the signs that precede death.

When a pregnant woman passes consecutively through these stages that end her life [and] dies, even now there is not enough certainty to proceed with the [cesarean operation]. Before doing this it is necessary to undertake further measures and to be alert to the signs that follow death.

When a pregnant woman's [health] worsens from one of these sicknesses, whether from weakness or irritation caused by a fever or from the convulsions that a miscarriage usually causes, one must be sure to take great care of the sick woman and baptize the fetus. The same care must be taken during her final death throes, because soon after the moment that she expires a miscarriage often follows, and the feto, forgotten under the clothing and bedcovers, would be suffocated and perhaps would not be baptized in time because the women, or the midwife, who are present with the dying woman do not use

15. According to the 1734 edition of the *Diccionario de autoridades* (vol. 4), *hética* is a sickness characterized by excessive heat and dryness in the body, along with an acidic stomach, night sweats, and weight loss. *Tipsca* is likely a variant of the word *tísico*, which means "tuberculosis" or "consumption." The author references different kinds of respiratory infections, the translations of which are lost to modern readers.

16. *Garrotillo* in the text referred to diphtheria. Cook and Lovell, *Secret Judgments of God*, 244.

their hands to check under the clothing and bedcovers, which must be carefully examined.

Also, we warn that when the sick woman finds herself very close to death, the attendants, the sick, or neighbors must notify the parish priest or the coadjutor that it is time to notify the surgeon or, if one is lacking, the barber-surgeon or whoever will conduct the operation. Likewise [notify] the alcaldes or Indigenous elites so that everyone can be ready. Place clear, warm water in a glass for the baptism. And if the criatura is in the later months [of development], prepare thick cloths to receive it and [call a] wet nurse.

Now everything is ready [so that] as soon as the woman dies according to the stages that I have described, she can immediately be covered. Remove the clothing and bedcovers from the bed, leaving the cadaver on it, or place it [the cadaver] on a table or on the floor on a *petate* in a place where there is sufficient light [17] Or, if it is night-time, place three lit candles [around the body].

Those present must now examine the body to see if it shows any indication of life. Carefully examine whether the heart and the senses beat or pulsate. Bring a light or a silver plate close to the nostrils and the mouth to see if there are any signs of respiration, taking care to ensure that there is no wind. Bring a lit [candle]wick to introduce smoke into the nostrils; yell loudly in the ears; place a heated rock or iron on the arm or the sole of the foot or on the head. If none of these actions cause a sign of life, if there is absolutely no pulse or respiration, [and] the body is heavy, cold, and stiff; the eyes dull and sunken; the nose gaunt; and the entire face has a deathly pallor, these are the signs that follow death, and at this point one can proceed with sufficient certainty with the operation.

[*Translated by Martha Few*]

Domingo Fajardo, "Petén Miscellanies," Gazeta de Guatemala, October 1, 1804, 453–54

[*In 1804 the* Gazeta de Guatemala, *the audiencia's newspaper, pub-lished a letter to the editor written by Domingo Fajardo, in which he described four postmortem cesarean operations that various men*

---

17. A *petate* is a traditional Mesoamerican-style woven mat made from plant leaves.

performed on deceased pregnant women in the Petén region. In the
colonial period this region consisted of a presidio and a series of
mission towns located along Lake Petén Itzá that were populated
primarily by Itzá and Kowoj Maya. During the late seventeenth
century, this area was the site of the conquest of the Itzá Maya, the
last independent Maya Kingdom. Though Spanish-led forces mili-
tarily defeated the Itzá, throughout the eighteenth century the lake
region remained a frontier zone. Fajardo's decision to send a letter
to the Gazeta de Guatemala *describing the cesareans that took place*
there shows how print media created opportunities for feedback.
News of the operations' performance recirculated the religious and
secular policy ideas that underpinned the spread of the postmortem
cesarean throughout the empire. Moreover, Fajardo's letter conveyed
how "this unknown corner of the world" nevertheless remained
connected to the larger eighteenth-century context by enacting the
operation.]

Support for the cesarean operation that Maestro Rodríguez so advocated for in his [essay] "Nuevo aspecto" and by others, including this
newspaper and even the *Gazeta de Madrid,* can also be found in this
unknown corner of the world. I have practiced it on the cadaver of
Damiana Montero, the wife of Felipe Navarrete. The presidio surgeon, Severino Luna, performed it and presented me with a criatura
who was baptized conditionally because she showed no signs of life.
Two minutes later I had the pleasure of seeing signs of life, then
she moved the fingers of one hand, gasped, and died on November
16, 1799. That was the date of her burial, as recorded in the parish
book with a note that the child had been extracted from the mother's
womb by cesarean operation.

In the town of San Andrés in this province, [the cesarean opera-
tion] was also performed by the presbyter Don Eusebio Villamíl, *cura*
reductor in the said town, on the cadaver of Dominga Chatá, Indian,
wife of Esteban Covoh, and the criatura was baptized conditionally
for not showing any signs of life.[18]

---

18. Reduction (*reducción*) was a Spanish colonial policy of forced resettlement of
native peoples into a model town for taxation and religious conversion. As *cura reduc-*
tor, Villamíl was a priest in charge of such a town.

A few months later a smallpox epidemic came to the said town, killing about half the residents, because it had been thirty years since it [i.e., the last smallpox epidemic] had been there. There were two pregnant women among the Indian women who died [from small-pox]. One of them was Juana May, wife of Pedro Batab. The said priest [Villamíl] performed the operation on her with such a good outcome, because the criatura [was] certified to be alive so that after the baptism, [the criatura then died and] was buried inside the church.

The other was Nicolasa Chatá, wife of Marcos Cob, of whom it is necessary to describe the heroism that she so willingly displayed, since among the Indians such highly uncommon religious sentiments are also found.

When Nicolasa was on the verge of death, the priest sent for the barber[-surgeon], who was Indian and who had been taught during the earlier operations, and he made the necessary preparations to perform the [cesarean]. The barber[-surgeon] unwisely placed the straight razor in the sick woman's room, where she saw it.[19] Then she called the priest, who was present in the house, and she begged him that because she had no hope of surviving, she feared that the criatura would die before she did. And because of this she was prepared to suffer the operation before her death, because then at least the criatura in her womb would not perish without baptism.

The priest did not dare, and he comforted her, saying that the feto would be cared for. A short time later the mother died. [The barber-surgeon] conducted the operation and successfully baptized the criatura, certain that it was alive, and, like the previous [one, it died and] was buried inside the church.

The first described case would have lost much of its believability if I had kept secret my name that was necessary to sanction [the operation]. That is why I say that it does not seem to me to be prudent to suppress it. I am your most attentive servant and clergyman who kisses your hand.

Domingo Faxardo
(Petén, July 11, 1804)

[Translated by Martha Few]

---

19. Referred to as *navaja barbero* and *navaja de barba*, the straight razor was used to conduct the cesarean operation.

Excerpts from Colonial New Spain

Ignacio Segura, Avisos saludables a las parteras para el cumplimiento de su obligación: Sacados de la embriología sacra del Sr. Dr. D. Francisco Manuel Cangiamila y puestos en castellano por el Dr. D. Ignacio Segura *(Mexico City: Zuñiga y Ontiveros, 1775), n.p. and 1, 2, 11–12, 23, 12, 19–20*

[*The work of Ignacio Segura, a physician in New Spain, resembles that of many other authors of cesarean operation treatises in that it borrows heavily from Cangiamila's* Sacred Embryology. *In addition, it twice directs readers to the more extensive translation of Cangiamila's work that José Manuel Rodríguez published in Mexico City under the title* La caridad del sacerdote para con los niños encerrados en el vientre de sus madres difuntas. *Segura's intended audience, however, was different from this and other published works. While most authors aimed to reach priests and other learned men through their writings, Segura was alone in focusing his efforts primarily on providing midwives with instruction in the operation. During the late colonial period, midwives assisted the vast majority of births in New Spain and elsewhere in the Spanish Empire. They were thus likely to be present when pregnant women died, and they could not necessarily count on securing the help of a knowledgeable surgeon or priest to perform the cesarean. Despite the fact that Segura expressed disdain for their competence, he argued that midwives should know how to carry out the operation and baptize. In his prologue Segura explained the relationship between his work and that of Cangiamila. He also conveyed concerns about the knowledge and skills of midwives in New Spain.*]

Having read the work of Dr. Cangiamila and used it to instruct myself in its many necessary points for doctors, it seemed to me that it would be useful to put into Spanish the warnings it contains regarding midwives. Some of these women are so poorly instructed, even in the most trivial issues, that their ignorance can be the cause of the bodily and spiritual death of many criaturas capable of both [temporal and spiritual] life, or at least the spiritual life. I consulted with knowledgeable and prudent people about my thinking. They approved, and thus I decided to give this small book to the clever superiors who profess medicine to make a compendium of the cited work, which I judge would be of great use to students and even to people further along in this and the other fields. Meanwhile, I dedicate this short work, in which I have invested, to the common benefit, the spiritual well-being of infants, and the growth of the triumphant and militant church.

[*Although Segura criticized midwives for their supposed ignorance, he saw them as crucial for fulfilling the church's goal of salvation through baptism.*]

The profession of the midwife is most useful for the health of the souls and of the bodies and even for the preservation of humankind, inasmuch it requires great charity and prudence. And for this reason they are called *wise women*, and *comothers*, as if they were second mothers for the infants.

[Midwives] are thus obligated under mortal sin to know how to baptize, seeking to preserve it [the instruction] in their memories. And if they forget anything or are in doubt, they should ask their priest. It will also be useful that they share this material and everything that is contained in this small book with the other women of their profession, and principally with those who seek to study it [midwifery].

[*Segura argued in his work that midwives should baptize only as a last resort.*]

In terms of the person who should baptize: although the baptism is always valid when administered with the due material, form, and intention, whether by a clergyman or a layperson, man or woman, Christian or infidel, it is nevertheless not always permissible for the midwife to baptize children, since they, by law, should be baptized in the church by the priest or vicar. Inasmuch, such midwives may perform it only in cases of extreme, or at the very least grave, risk of death for the criatura and when there is no other Christian, not even a layperson, who might know and be able to baptize it.

[*Segura provided instructions regarding the appropriate waters for use in baptism by midwives. Some of these differed from those Arrese listed in his work.*]

The material for the baptism is natural water—that is to say, rainwater, [or] water from the sea, from rivers or from springs or from wells. Be advised that when the midwife baptizes, or another person does so in case it is needed, it is not necessary that the water be blessed, nor that it be salty or have salt added to it. It is convenient that the midwife have clean water prepared for her in an earthenware bowl, from which she will draw for the endangered criaturas, who have not been born, and in a jug, which is for the purpose of the baptism of those already born. But she cannot use artificial waters such as rosewater, orange blossom water, or others, unless it is the case that natural water is totally lacking, and in such a case one should state this condition: *if I can with this water.* If there is natural water [available] afterward, she should baptize again with this condition: *if you are not baptized.* The water should be poured on the head in such a way that it touches the flesh and runs across it. Pour it three times, making with each one a sign of the cross.

[*Segura believed midwives also needed instruction in the cesarean operation.*]

If, upon opening the belly of the deceased when pregnancy is certain, the criatura does not appear, open the belly somewhat more deeply and look for it with great care, because it may have been conceived outside of the womb. In order to understand this, you should instruct yourselves as much as possible in the art of childbirth, either learning from some book that touches on this or asking the most intelligent surgeons or attending anatomical dissections carried out on women. If you, principally the novices, do not carry out one of these diligences, you will commit a thousand errors.

If one time instead of a criatura you find a fleshy mass or a false monstrosity, you should open it, because sometimes one finds criaturas within them. Therefore, in the cesarean birth or when women expel such fleshy masses, you should open all of them, even in the case when a criatura also came out. And be advised that it is safest to open with one's fingers whenever possible, so as not to risk cutting the criatura if one does it with a knife.

[*Among his critiques of midwives, Segura expressed little faith in their ability to judge whether a fetus was dead before or during the birthing process.*]

It is most appropriate to warn midwives not to be mistaken, believing that the stench caused by the mother's corrupted humors is caused by the corruption of the criatura and thus taking it for dead. They should also know that gangrene is one thing and corruption of the dead something else. Among other signs one identifies gangrene, whether dry or moist, when one finds a rubicund, or good-looking, color at the end of said gangrene, and there the healthy part is separated off from the gangrenous. At the same time being born bruised stems most often from the constriction the criatura suffers upon leaving: with which it is not always due to putrefaction.

[*Segura also doubted midwives' judgments with regard to births considered at the time to be "monstrous," meaning that the offspring did not resemble how a newborn was expected to appear in its physical form.*]

It is illicit to kill a criatura, even though it may be excessively ugly or monstrous. And thus, if time allows, they should call the priest so that he can determine whether the monster should be baptized. But if the danger [of dying] is very urgent, they will baptize it promptly, in accordance with the rules we have given. Dwarves, hunchbacks, and similar [criaturas] are usually full of life, but the excessively horrific criaturas do not usually live long. In any case it is illicit to kill them, even after baptizing them.

[*Translated by Adam Warren*]

[*The series of excerpts that follow—all taken from the late colonial newspaper* Gazeta de México—*are typical in that they describe postmortem cesareans performed primarily, though not exclusively, on Indigenous women. These print references are simultaneously mundane yet extraordinary, not least for the details that they shed on prevalent ideas surrounding childbirth, gender, medical knowledge, the animation of the soul, fetal baptism, and death. We have uncovered references, between the years of 1794 and 1826, to some thirteen postmortem cesarean operations in several newspaper entries, of which we have included a number. The entry published on June 20, 1795, is one of the rare accounts we have of the postmortem cesarean being performed on a Spanish woman.*]

Excerpt from Gazeta de México, *January 21, 1795*

Panotlán, December 30 [1794]
Over the course of the past five years in this curate there were 326 marriages, 944 baptisms, and 529 burials. Of those who had been baptized, four have achieved this [eternal] happiness by benefit of the cesarean operation, performed twice with the necessary precautions by the parish priest Dr. Don Urbano Antonio Díaz de las Cuevas;

another by one of his vicars, Don Francisco Álvarez; and the other by Don Joachín Torres, surgeon and resident of Tlaxcala.

[*Translated by Zeb Tortorici*]

Excerpt from Gazeta de México, June 20, 1795

Chiautla de la Sal, June 1 [1795].
On the twentieth of April, in this *cabecera* of Chiautla de la Sal, Brígada Ruiz, who was married to Miguel de Leon, both Spaniards, died.[20] As a result of having received notice that she was five months pregnant, the subdelegate mandated that the cesarean operation be carried out. [And through the operation] it was achieved that the girl, who was about the size of a *tercia*, came out alive, and after some time she died.[21]

[*Translated by Zeb Tortorici*]

Excerpt from Gazeta de México, May 29, 1799

Mission of Santa Clara in Nueva California, January 26 [1799].
The reverend fathers Friar Joseph Viader and Friar Joseph Viñals verified the cesarean operation on a pregnant Indian woman of eight months, according to the records, who was weakened by a violent typhus fever. Their ignorance of anatomy, their lack of medical books, and their never having seen a similar operation performed were not sufficient to frighten them in their envisioned enterprise: all of this would seem to bode poorly, though accompanied by an effective desire to eternally unite with God the criatura, who otherwise would forcibly perish in sin, [which] made them overcome all obstacles. By the forces of evil, the neophyte died on the day of the birth and immediately after the operation was performed, the success of which surpassed all expectations of the fathers, who demonstrated their consummate joy in baptizing the extracted boy with much less effort than they confusedly expected. Even the most scrupulous decency would not resent having attended the operation. And although the most conducive diligences were practiced aimed at his preservation, given that the mother during her illness could not nourish him, nor

---

20. A *cabecera* is an administrative center of a political jurisdiction.
21. A *tercia* is a measure of length, approximately eleven inches.

could anyone else, he survived only seven hours after the operation. We extend this notice so that the many criaturas in all similar cases do not become the victims of irresolution and fear, for through this means they can acquire eternal happiness.[22]

[*Translated by Zeb Tortorici*]

Excerpt from Gazeta de México, *November 11, 1799*

Mission of San Antonio de Oquitoa in the Pimería Alta, Province of Sonora, September 26, [17]98.

Maria Antonia Zapatito, wife of Christobal Bravo, Indians of this mission, died there on the [aforementioned] date. She was five or six months pregnant, and the missionary father Friar Ramón López, desiring to aid the feto with the holy baptism, fearing the proximate death of the mother, and entrusted by God with the wise choice of [performing] the operation demanded by the circumstances in a country lacking trained medical doctors and other assistants, readied the midwife and Francisco López de Xérez, retired sergeant of the Presidio del Altar Company, so that they became the operation's agents under the instructions of the watchful Cangiamila in his *Sacred Embryology.*

[After] the said minister and the others present verified the death of the aforementioned woman, the sergeant proceeded to open the right side with a barber's knife, having prepared a bucket of water immediately next to the cadaver. And [after he finished] cutting all the teguments with fortunate success, the midwife then introduced her hands into the womb. And in a short time of two minutes, she extracted the afterbirth, or pouch, with the criatura enveloped within it. It was immediately baptized, surviving eight minutes afterward.[23]

In another case of the same type involving the wife of the soldier Manuel Moreno, Ignacia Martinez, who was pregnant for eight

22. "Misión de Santa Clara en la Nueva California," *Gazeta de México,* May 29, 1799; "Fr. Joseph Viader y Fr. Joseph Viñals acordaron verificar la operación cesárea en una India preñada, segun indicios, de ocho meses, postrada de un violento tabardillo," *Gazeta de México,* January 26, 1799. Given their ignorance of anatomy, lack of books, and inexperience in similar operations, they did not succeed. Reid, "Medics of the Soul," 100, gives the archival reference for this case: death record, Santa Clara (SCL) 02218, Early California Population Project Database, Huntington Library, San Marino.

23. Afterbirth, or "pouch," is *zurrón* in the original, which refers to the amniotic sac.

months, Father Francisco Moyano was pleased with himself for having successfully executed the previously mentioned said cesarean operation about three hours after she died. She was already shrouded and laid out in the home at the time that the aforementioned missionary, who came to confess her, arrived from Oquitoa.

Those who performed the procedure were the same [people] mentioned previously; they extracted the criatura alive, which survived a half hour after receiving the baptism, with great consolation of its relatives, [who] only some time earlier had resisted the practice of the operation, perhaps for having not heard about it or for believing it attributable only to medical doctors.

Both of these cases are presented [here in the *Gazeta de México*] so that by spreading their news, the zeal of the parish priests will be roused in favor of the souls of similar criaturas, and they will seek to learn the means of practicing the operation, by which means they [the priests] can make them eternally blessed. And [since] this is one of the matters most worthy of attention, it has seemed opportune to repeat the warning that Dr. and Maestro Joseph García Jove, *protomédico* in this capital [Mexico City], gave. He warned that while the *Gazeta of Goatemala* [sic] fundamentally promoted the care that must be taken in similar cases, and in those of difficult births or miscarriages, to rupture the afterbirth or [amniotic] sac with which the infants are enveloped in the mother's womb, if one were to proceed to baptize them without this precaution, the fruit of this sacrament would be denied, and they would remain unbaptized, since not they, but rather the sac, is that which receives the [holy] water.

[*Translated by Zeb Tortorici*]

Vicente Francisco de Sarría, "Operación cesárea y misioneros de California,"
1830, BANC MSS C-C 26, Bancroft Library (University of California, Berkeley)

[*Vicente Francisco de Sarría (1767–1835) was born in Spain, where he joined the Franciscan order. Although few details exist about his life, we know that he traveled to New Spain as a missionary priest in 1804 and ended up in Alta California in 1809, where he was assigned as parish priest to the missions San Carlos (1809–29) and Soledad (1829–35). After reading Antonio José Rodríguez's* Nuevo aspecto de teología médico-moral, *he wrote a letter to those in charge of the missions in Alta California, from the mission of San Carlos to San*

*Francisco Solano, spreading information about the religious impor-
tance of performing postmortem cesareans for fetal baptism.*]

Hail Jesus, Mary, and Joseph

Most Reverend Apostolic Fathers from Mission San Carlos to that of
San Francisco Solano.

My most beloved fathers and sirs—health and peace to you all
in the name of Jesus Christ. I have still not seen any notice nor any
public paper at all concerning our ministry, of which I am a member
by the grace of our Lord, that addresses or even touches on in the
slightest the cesarean operation.

Nevertheless, familiarity with [the operation] is so important for
the possible cases, in which the salvation of souls depends on its regular providence.[24] And since personal and domestic examples move
one to be persuaded *more effectively*, I will provide a single case in
an effort to prove my point. From the work of the reverend father
Cistercian monk Antonio José Rodríguez, titled *Nuevo aspecto de
teología médico-moral y ambos derechos*, where, among many other
matters, that illustrious author addresses fundamentally and scientif-
ically the cesarean operation, one learns that one of those who have
promoted the operation the most in recent years for opening the
doors of eternal salvation to miscarried children has been not just a
member of our seraphic profession but one engaged in the work of an
apostolic missionary. The book results from what he saw in reference
to it during the course of his missions.

Since it is worthy of some notice on our part, I will convey what
the aforementioned author presents in this respect in the fourth volume of his cited work, paradox 1, marginal number 24.

And, for the sake of the same, I will add that in the year of
1760, when I was approving, in Madrid, the revision and licens-
ing of my books, the learned and pious father Friar Deodato
de Cúneo, observant priest [of the religious orders], published
in Venice a volume dedicated to the salvation of the unborn
and the aborted. Filled with the spirit of charity and love of his

24. Here "providence" refers to anticipation and preparation.

fellow man, he assured that he was moved to write this work, on the baptism of fetos and the opening [up] of deceased mothers to help the child with baptism, because of the repeated experiences of the innumerable loss of souls due to the carelessness of abortions [miscarriages], which he learned of and saw in the course of his missionary work.

Thus far [speaks] the illustrious Cistercian, and he also adds that this neglect and the love that he had [in] attending to this remedy made such an impression on his soul (that is, of the devout missionary about whom he speaks here) that in order to attend to every [case], he deliberately studied all there is, according to what is seen in his book, and he can guarantee the safety of his project. In various other passages of his treatise [*Nuevo aspecto*], he also cites with particular respect that good father and missionary.

And since it is not believed among the faithful that these cases are very rare, even when speaking of the missions, allow me to convey what happened to me in the few trips I took to them while finding myself in our apostolic school, before moving to them [i.e., the missions].

A pregnant woman died near the village where we carried out our mission (it is called Coatepeq). She confessed, it appears to me, shortly before dying, as far as I recall, having been summoned and gone to her. [After she] passed away in this manner, and with the priest absent from the parish where we were, another priest from among those who carried out the mission and I got ourselves ready to undertake the operation, based on the obligation we perceived ourselves to have in this case. And not finding an apt subject in whom to entrust [the operation's performance], we picked up the book that discussed it so that, with one reading its respective contents and the other carrying it out word for word, we might perform the work ourselves.

However, at this moment the midwife, or birth assistant, an older woman who seemed experienced in her profession, came and spoke with us. She assured us that the criatura was dead for a reason or reasons that she gave us, [reasons] with which I now disagree, but which we took at the time as sufficient to believe her and cease the operation, as we in fact did.

If the case were to happen again now, after having read Father Rodríguez in his aforementioned work, the *Nuevo aspecto de teología médico-moral, etc.*, I would surely not be assuaged, and while able I would take steps to carry out [the operation].

After bringing in the most revealing testimonies of distinguished physicians in their profession and even of Protestant authors to prove that one should not neglect to open any woman who dies while pregnant, the aforementioned Father Rodríguez referred to the case of the surgeon Hyldmo, who admitted to having been deceived. He believed the feto to be dead but nevertheless continued operating on the mother as much as needed to show that it had died. It was extracted alive and did not die until the third day. Rodríguez then confirms this with another notable example:

> But still (these are his words on page 26 of volume 4 of the previously specified work) it is even more urgent for the disillusion in the case that transpired before the same Cangiamila in October 1736. A poor, young woman of the same parish [as he] died in the state of pregnancy. The midwife, who was mature in her profession, and the surgeon, who was famous and had practiced in the hospital of Sancti Spiritus [the Holy Ghost] in Rome, attested to and assured without any doubt that the feto had already died two days prior to [the death of] its mother. Nothing assuaged Cangiamila; he had the deceased opened, and he took out a live girl, who was baptized with the name of Placida, and she lived a quarter of an hour. The learned and pious ecclesiastic wanted to fully carry out his triumph. He buried the girl with much ceremony, officiating the burial himself, an act that caused great spiritual joy for the entire town.

Such is what the celebrated Cistercian author writes in the *Nuevo aspecto de teología, etc.*, which in truth is no longer so new, since as we saw before in his statement, the revisions were being carried out in the year 60 of the previous century in order to send this work to the press.

The adjoining practical instructions for the cesarean operation are taken almost entirely from what I have seen (none of it comes from me, but rather from having made a copy that accompanies the earlier ones) of what the same author [Rodríguez] describes, which is said to be according to the teachings of the best surgeons and especially the French surgeon Francisco [François] Mauriceau, who practiced the obstetric arts for forty years in Paris. Also, (they say) Monsignor Cangiamila and the aforementioned our Father Deodato describe it as well, but he [Rodríguez] thinks Mauriceau's instructions are preferable because of his great experience.

I barely have breath to speak to Your Reverences about the issue of making copies of it [the instructions], because I know very well the difficulties and hindrances among so many other matters needing attention within our ministry. But, I would like that, following the obligations of charity, my fathers not allow a soul to perish, being mindful of what the goal is and considering that a case [of a pregnant woman's death] might arise when one least imagines it, and that in a mission it cannot fail to happen as part of the normal course of events, especially if one has the diligence of knowing whether or not a woman who dies at the proportionate age and disposition [for pregnancy] has a feto in her womb. And so the resource for that moment is a practical, clear, and easy set of guidelines, which is what I present. I would like that Your Reverences, drawing on the ardor of your zeal and nature for the best fulfillment of your duties, make a brief effort in this case, copying or having a copy made of what is joined together here, unless there is already another approved work or book in the mission that addresses the same topic in particular. [It must] belong to the mission so that [priests] might never be without these practical guidelines, and it will govern when it is necessary or convenient to perform the cesarean operation.

It is not enough for this effort that the father minister who serves his mission know or have experience in carrying it out without needing further instruction, since after him another one will follow, who, according to the chances of our good ministerial fortune, might not know it. Beyond the possibility that the most learned [priest] may find something that interests him in the various pettiness and trivialities that are made present in this work, for the best and most happy [readers], it gives them what is desired.

So that one may make the aforementioned copy, which, as Your Reverences see, I especially recommend to you, you may hold onto the notice, whether for eight or ten days, and thereby take whatever space is convenient for it. And for the same [notice] and to not delay on the issue too long, I have procured to make copies such that one may go from here to Santa Barbara and may circulate until that point

along the way among the intermediate missions in the regular manner. Another sent immediately to San Buenaventura should circulate
successively from there as far as San Diego and another at the same
time as that one from the missions around here to San Francisco
Solano.

Having signed below sequentially, you shall return it from the last
mission previously *named* with the accompanying copy.

It is in the union of Your Reverences' prayers and holy sacrifices
in beautiful and fervent ministry in the name of our Lord, may he
protect you many years.

[Mission] Nuestra Señora de la Soledad
July 26, 1830

Friar Vicente Francisco de Sarría

Despite pertaining to the library of Mission San Carlos the work of
the Cistercian reverend father Antonio José Rodríguez, from which
the instructions for the cesarean operation were copied, I will copy
this advisory, from which the reverend father Friar Antonio Menén-
dez has copied. This advisory has been held for many days, and
because I arrived beforehand it is not me who delayed it.

San Juan Bautista
August 19, 1830
Friar Ramón Abesta

San Juan Bautista and August 19, 1830

I am ordered to return with consideration for now the instructions
for the cesarean operation, and I have complied.

Friar Felipe Arroyo de la Cuesta

Santa Cruz, August 28, 1830

I have copied (as the reverend father prefect orders) the cesarean operation.

Friar Juan Moreno

Santa Clara, September 2, 1830

The cesarean operation has been copied.

Friar José Méndez

San José, September 3 [1830]

I have copied the way to perform the cesarean operation.

Friar Narciso Durán

Mission of San Francisco, September 8, 1830

The cesarean operation is being copied.

Friar Thomas Estenaga

San Rafael Arcángel, September 30, 1830

The treatise or way to perform the cesarean operation has been copied.

Friar Juan Amorás

San Francisco Solano, October 12, 1830

The treatise on the cesarean operation has been copied from the initial part where it begins: *Repeated thanks* until the end where it concludes: *You will be a helper to the orphan.*[25]

Friar Buenav. Fortuna
[*Translated by Adam Warren and Zeb Tortorici*][26]

---

25. The original sentence is in Latin.
26. A portion of this excerpt was previously translated by Cook, in "Sarria's Treatise," 107–9.

aborto. A miscarried or aborted fetus. Biological material expelled during a miscarriage.

audiencia. A territory that falls under the jurisdiction of a royal high court in the Spanish Empire. In Spain's American colonies, each viceroyalty was jurisdictionally divided into multiple audiencias.

Audiencia of Guatemala A royal court that exercised jurisdiction over what is today Guatemala, Honduras, El Salvador, Belize, Nicaragua, Costa Rica, and the Mexican state of Chiapas. It was part of the Viceroyalty of New Spain

bando. A published edict or a mandate issued by governmental authorities.

barber-surgeon. An informal medical practitioner who performed his work primarily with the use of a razor and practiced minor forms of surgery. The procedures that barber-surgeons performed included, but were not limited to, bloodletting, pulling teeth, and cupping. Barber-surgeons also provided services such as shaving, trimming facial hair, cutting hair, and bathing.

catechism. A summary of the basic tenets of Christianity in the form of questions and answers, used for the instruction of Christians.

conditional baptism. The performance of the ritual of baptism when the fetus's life is in doubt. It usually includes language indicating that the sacrament's validity depends on whether the fetus in question is alive.

criatura. Child, infant, or fetus. Like the term *feto,* as used in the eighteenth century, it could refer to a fetus or newborn located either inside or outside the womb.

curia diocesana. A group of persons who assist the bishop of that diocese.

embryology. The branches of medicine and, in this case, religion concerned with the study of embryos and their development.

entierro doble. "Double burial," which refers to the burial of a deceased pregnant woman and her deceased fetus (as often recorded in parish death records or burial registries), after their deaths during childbirth or due to a postmortem cesarean operation.

feto. Fetus. During the eighteenth century a feto could in practice be located in the womb, be recently born, or be surgically extracted from the womb through postmortem cesarean operation.

gazeta.   The term for newspapers in the eighteenth century that circulated throughout the Spanish Empire. These newspapers are crucial sources in that they recorded dozens, if not hundreds, of postmortem cesareans.

holy sacraments.   The necessary religious ceremonies of the Christian church regarded as outward and visible signs of divine grace. The seven sacraments are baptism, Eucharist, confirmation, penance, anointing of the sick, holy orders, and matrimony.

limbo.   In Catholic theology an intermediary space on the edge of hell where unbaptized infants and others exist.

mestizo.   An individual of mixed Indigenous and European heritage.

mission.   A religious outpost, usually on the fringes of a Spanish colonial territory, in which members of Catholic religious orders—largely Franciscans, Dominicans, and Jesuits—engaged in evangelizing the region's Indigenous populations.

partera.   Midwife. The Latin term for the midwife was *obstetrix*, sometimes written in Spanish as *obstetriz*.

pragmática.   A royal proclamation, several of which were issued regarding postmortem cesarean operations. The first such cesarean-related pragmática, issued by Charles III on August 9, 1749, required the operation's performance and the baptism of the unborn in the Kingdom of Sicily; this *pragmática* eventually applied to Spain and its overseas colonies.

presbyter.   A priest or minister of the Catholic Church.

presidio.   A Spanish colonial fort and outpost, often located on the fringes of the Spanish Empire in conjunction with missions.

promotor fiscal.   A prosecuting officer (in ecclesiastical, inquisitorial, or diocesan courts) trained in civil and canon law.

reducción.   A centralized village of Indigenous inhabitants created through the Spanish colonial policy of forced resettlement of native peoples (also known as *congregación*).

viceroyalty.   A vast territorial and administrative unit administered by a viceroy. The Spanish Americas were initially divided into two viceroyalties—of New Spain (officially established in 1535 and encompassing Mexico, Central America, Florida, much of the southwestern and central United States, the Caribbean, and eventually the Philippines) and of Peru (established in 1542 and including what is today South America, with the exception of Brazil). Later reforms established the Viceroyalty of New Granada in 1717 (including what is today largely Panama, Venezuela, Ecuador, and Colombia) and, in 1776, the Viceroyalty of the Río de la Plata (including what is today largely Argentina, Bolivia, Paraguay, and Uruguay).

zamba.   An individual of mixed Indigenous and African parentage.

Arrese, Pedro José de. *Rudimentos físico, canónico, morales . . . sobre el bautismo de fetos abortivos y operación cesárea en las mugeres, que mueren embarazadas.* Guatemala City: Viuda de Arévalo, 1786.

Bernard de Gordon. *Practica sive lilium medicinae.* Lyons, 1498.

Blumenfeld-Kosinski, Renate. *Not of Woman Born: Representations of Caesarean Birth in Medieval and Renaissance Culture.* Ithaca: Cornell University Press, 1990.

Bouley, Bradford A. *Pious Postmortems: Anatomy, Sanctity, and the Catholic Church in Early Modern Europe.* Philadelphia: University of Pennsylvania Press, 2017.

Brind'Amour, Katherine. "Quickening." *Embryo Project Encyclopedia.* October 30, 2007. https://embryo.asu.edu/pages/quickening.

Cangiamila, Francisco [Francesco]. *Embriología sagrada, ó tratado de la obligación que tienen los curas, confesores, médicos, comadres, y otras personas, de cooperar á la salvación de los niños que aun no han nacido, de los que nacen al parecer muertos, de los abortivos, de los monstruos, etc.* Vol. 2. Translated by Joaquín Castellot. Madrid: Imprenta de Marin, 1774.

Caulhiaco, Guigonis de [Guy de Chauliac]. *Inventarium sive Chirurgia Magna.* Vol. 1. Edited by Michael R. McVaugh. Leiden: Brill, 1997.

Cook, Noble David, and William George Lovell, eds. *"Secret Judgments of God": Old World Disease in Colonial Spanish America.* Norman: University of Oklahoma Press, 1992.

Cook, Sherburne F. "Sarria's Treatise on the Cesarean Operation, 1830." *California and Western Medicine* 47, no. 2 (1937): 107–9; 47, no. 3 (1937): 187–89; 47, no. 4 (1937): 248–50.

Demerson, Paula de. "La cesárea *post mortem* en la España de la Ilustración." *Ascelpio* 28 (1976): 185–233.

Diccionario de autoridades. Vol. 3. Madrid: Real Academia Española, 1732.

———— . Vol. 4. Madrid: Real Academia Española, 1734.

———— . Vol. 5. Madrid: Real Academia Española, 1737.

Dym, Jordana. "Conceiving Central America: A Bourbon Public in the Gazeta de Guatemala (1797–1807)." In *Enlightened Reform in Southern Europe and Its Atlantic Colonies, c. 1750–1850,* edited by Gabriel Paquette, 99–118. Burlington, Vt.: Ashgate, 2009.

Few, Martha. *For All of Humanity: Mesoamerican and Colonial Medicine in Enlightenment Guatemala*. Tucson: University of Arizona Press, 2015.
———. *Women Who Live Evil Lives: Gender, Religion, and the Politics of Power in Colonial Guatemala*. Austin: University of Texas Press, 2002.

Hopwood, Nick, Rebecca Flemming, and Lauren Kassell, eds. *Reproduction: Antiquity to the Present Day*. Cambridge: Cambridge University Press, 2019.

Jaffary, Nora E. *Reproduction and Its Discontents in Mexico: Childbirth and Contraception from 1750 to 1905*. Chapel Hill: University of North Carolina Press, 2016.

Lanning, John Tate. *The Eighteenth-Century Enlightenment in the University of San Carlos de Guatemala*. Ithaca: Cornell University Press, 1956.

Navas, Juan de. *Elementos del arte de partear*. Pt. 2. Madrid: Imprenta Real, 1795.

Park, Katharine. "Managing Childbirth and Fertility in Medieval Europe." In Hopwood, Flemming, and Kassell, *Reproduction*, 153–66.

Real Academia Española. *Diccionario de la lengua castellana compuesto por la Real Academia Española, reducido a un tomo para su más fácil uso*. Madrid: Ibarra, 1780.

Reid, Anne Marie. "Medics of the Soul and the Body: Sickness and Death in Alta California, 1769–1850." PhD diss., University of Southern California, 2013.

Rigau-Pérez, José G. "Surgery at the Service of Theology: Postmortem Cesarean Sections in Puerto Rico and the Royal Cédula of 1804." *Hispanic American Historical Review* 75, no. 3 (1995): 377–404.

Rodríguez, Antonio Joseph [José]. *Nuevo aspecto de teología médico-moral, y ambos derechos, ó paradoxas físico-teológico legales: Obra crítica, provechoso á párrocos, confesores, y profesores de ambos derechos, y útil a médicos, filósofos y eruditos*. Vol. 4. 3rd ed. Madrid: Imprenta de Cano, 1787.

Turner, Sasha. *Contested Bodies: Pregnancy, Childrearing, and Slavery in Jamaica*. Philadelphia: University of Pennsylvania Press, 2017.

Valle, Rosemary Keupper. "The Cesarean Operation in Alta California During the Franciscan Mission Period (1769–1833)." *Bulletin of the History of Medicine* 48, no. 2 (1974): 265–75.

Van der Lugt, Maaike. "Formed Fetuses and Healthy Children in Scholastic Theology." In Hopwood, Flemming, and Kassell, *Reproduction*, 167–80.

Ventura Pastor, José. *Preceptos generales sobre las operaciones de los partos*. Madrid: Herrera, 1790.

Warren, Adam. "An Operation for Evangelization: Friar Francisco González Laguna, the Cesarean Section, and Fetal Baptism in Late Colonial Peru." *Bulletin of the History of Medicine* 83, no. 4 (2009): 647–75.

Wellmann, Janina. *The Form of Becoming: Embryology and the Epistemology of Rhythm, 1760–1830*. New York: Zone Books, 2017.